Mature Sexual Intimacy

Mature Sexual Intimacy

Making Menopause a
Turning Point, Not an Ending

Maryann Karinch

ROWMAN & LITTLEFIELD
Lanham • Boulder • New York • London

Published by Rowman & Littlefield
An imprint of The Rowman & Littlefield Publishing Group, Inc.
4501 Forbes Boulevard, Suite 200, Lanham, Maryland 20706
www.rowman.com

6 Tinworth Street, London SE11 5AL, United Kingdom

British Library Cataloguing in Publication Information Available

Library of Congress Cataloging-in-Publication Data
Names: Karinch, Maryann, author.
Title: Mature sexual intimacy : making menopause a turning point not an
  ending / Maryann Karinch.
Description: Lanham : Rowman & Littlefield, [2019] | Includes bibliographical
  references and index.
Identifiers: LCCN 2018053697 (print) | LCCN 2018058653 (ebook) | ISBN
  9781538113967 (Electronic) | ISBN 9781538113950 (cloth)
Subjects: LCSH: Menopause—Popular works. | Menopause—Physiological aspects.
  | Sex. | Women—Health and hygiene.
Classification: LCC RG186 (ebook) | LCC RG186 .K3727 2019 (print) | DDC
  618.1/75—dc23
LC record available at https://lccn.loc.gov/2018053697

To my loving partner, Jim McCormick

Contents

Acknowledgments

Two men figure very prominently into my acknowledgments because I would not be here without their partnership and caring: my dearest partner, Jim McCormick, and my amazing physician and co-author of *Sex and Cancer*, Saketh Guntupalli.

I owe tremendous thanks to the physicians, medical device and personal products experts, sex therapists, physical therapists, sex and sensual researchers, and nutritionists who generously contributed their insights, as well as to the people supporting them who provided documents and background information that was vital to making the discussions accurate (in alphabetical order): Betsy Cairo, PhD, HCLD, CSE, CSES, executive director, Look Both Ways, Inc. (www.lkbthwys.org); Carolyn Dean, MD ND, on the medical board of the nonprofit Nutritional Magnesium Association and author of *Menopause Naturally* and *The Magnesium Miracle* (second edition, 2017); Rebecca Dunsmoor-Su, MD, MSCE, FACOG, owner, RENUvaGYN, and director of health, genneve.com; Alyssa Dweck, MS, MD, FACOG, voted a "Top Doctor" in *New York Magazine* and medical advisor for menopause symptom-reliever Relizen; Rachel Gelman, DPT, PT, branch director, Pelvic Health and Rehabilitation Center, San Francisco; Suzan French Gennace, president of FlackShack; Mallory Junggren, senior director of Marketing JDS Therapeutics, LLC; Lori Ann King, wellness expert and author of *Come Back Strong*; Boris Levitsky, Net Improvements; Trevor Crow Mullineaux, LMFT, author of *Forging Healthy Connections* and *Blending Families*; Shannon Perry, director of media and

ix

marketing, genneve.com; Carol Queen, PhD, Good Vibrations Staff Sexologist; Brent Reider, designer of Yarlap and six other Class II medical devices cleared by the Food and Drug Administration as well as in Europe; Jenni Skyler, PhD, LMFT, CST, founder of The Intimacy Institute of Boulder and originator of the Cheesecake of Pleasure; C. Nicole ("Doc") Swiner, MD, a family physician voted #1 of 10 Best Doctors in North Carolina in 2017, and author of *How to Avoid the Superwoman Complex*; Beverly Whipple, PhD, RN, FAAN, professor emerita, Rutgers University, author of *Safe Encounters* and *The G Spot* and five other books, and the researcher who identified and named the G spot with her colleague John Perry as part of their teaching pelvic muscle contractions to women to treat urinary stress incontinence; Robert S. Wool, MD, co-founder of Women's Health Associates and a thirty-year veteran in quality women's health; and Yvonne Wray, computer scientist and an instructor with The Welcomed Consensus.

Speaking of The Welcomed Consensus, I want to thank my amazing client Ginger Testerman, whose parents founded this great teaching organization focused on women's pleasure. Anyone who finds this book useful should (please) visit their website (www.welcomed.com) and prepare to learn as well as enjoy a new level of intimacy.

Thank you, once again, to my editor, Suzanne Staszak-Silva, and to Hannah Fisher and the rest of the outstanding Rowman & Littlefield team. Working with you is a joy and a privilege!

I also want to thank so many friends, whom I believe would like to remain anonymous so their disclosures are not associated with them. You know who you are and how much you gave me. We are all women of a certain, exciting age with amazing relationships that naturally go up and down and up and up—with the "up" being intimacy that has gone from a boil to a steady, satisfying simmer and back to an occasional boil! Thank you specifically to my friends in the PEO sisterhood and my best gal pals from college who chat about all kinds of things with me as part of my "research."

Last but not least, I want to thank my dear mother, Ann Karinch, and my brother, Karl Karinch, who stand by me in all these investigations and products of my curious brain. I love you.

Introduction

Why This Book Is for All Women

What if you were a man wandering around at a cocktail party and found yourself abutting a small group of women chatting about something in an animated way. You innocently ask what's being discussed. One of the women says, "Dry vaginas."

That's exactly the scenario described in an article called "The Menopausal Vagina Monologues" that appeared in the *New York Times* on September 3, 2018. Dr. Randi Hutter Epstein, the physician who wrote the piece, wanted to make the point that vaginal dryness, or vaginal atrophy, is an extremely common problem for women in menopause, yet "less than half of those women seek help."[1]

This book is meant to be part of the "help"—a private way of exploring improved sexual health and science-based answers to finding physical comfort and pleasure during and after menopause. And I mean "comfort and pleasure" in all forms, from menopause symptom relief to orgasm.

In conversing with many women aged between forty-five and eighty-five years, I asked about their sexual activity. To me, a surprising number of women in the middle of that age range—mid-fifties to mid-sixties—indicated that they had little or no sex life. These are women with spouses or long-time partners. Many of them didn't even think masturbation was worth their time and energy.

If I were a character in the Sunday comics, the balloon above my head would have said, "Don't you think more of yourself than that?" I didn't say that out loud, of course.

Are you pushing back now, wishing I could hear your miffed tone as you ask, "What do you mean by that?"

I mean this: Respecting your humanity involves having desires and fulfilling them. Many of those desires reflect what your body and mind need to stay active, enjoy your day, cope with stress, battle sickness, feel competent, and so on. You want professional recognition, so you prepare diligently for each meeting to make sure you get it. You allow yourself to fantasize about a yummy mocha latte and then walk to the coffee shop to make your dream come true. You want to be healthy so you drag yourself to the gym; the desire to be in good shape overpowers your essential dislike of jogging on a treadmill.

You also want a loving touch. All human beings who are not seriously dysfunctional want a loving touch. Why wouldn't you want that loving touch to come from your life partner—and on a regular basis?

You deserve the physical satisfaction of intimacy. You deserve to know what to do to have that satisfaction. This book is about the value of intimacy, the rewards of it, and how to move yourself toward those rewards when you are perimenopausal or in the throes of menopause, or have emerged on the other side of it.

I urge you to think highly enough of yourself to say out loud, "I deserve pleasure."

It's apparently quite common for couples to choose a sexless life together, or for one to prefer that and the other to simply go along with the program. The label for this is companionate love, and it means you have everything you need to sustain a long-term relationship, but passion is not present.

This book is not a criticism of companionate love. It is, however, an invitation to every reader to at least browse through the reasons why sexual intimacy in our mature years is worth investing time and energy in—as well as the guidance on how to do that.

I have had the great privilege of interviewing some of the most extraordinary sex researchers, sensual researchers, and sexual health experts of our time for this book. They took my understanding of sexuality and sexual intimacy to new heights. Through this book, I want you to join me on top of the mountain and enjoy the panoramic view of our possibilities for achieving satisfying intimacy in our mature years.

Even if you never want to have sex again, the information in this book is, in many ways, useful to you.

A lab technician at our local hospital told me something I'll never forget that illustrates my point. After having unusual bleeding, my gynecologist ordered a transvaginal ultrasound to determine the cause. Transvaginal means "through the vagina." Making me laugh, relax, and listen, she explained how and why she would insert a wand into the vaginal canal and then take pictures. I was comfortable with the procedure, but asked her if anyone had ever been really upset by it.

"Yes," she said. "Usually it's fear of what we might find, but one patient couldn't handle the procedure itself." The woman found the ultrasound traumatic because she said it was the first time anything had been inserted there since she'd stopped seeing a gynecologist twenty years before. It was also painful due to vaginal atrophy. She was a seventy-year-old nun.

Even a vow of celibacy is not an excuse for ignoring vaginal health, a key theme in this book. Total physical and mental health means taking care of yourself from top to bottom.

Some of the advice from experts that can help you have an enjoyable sex life will also alleviate incontinence and eliminate the pain of a pelvic exam, among other benefits. A psychological benefit is feeling a little younger.

Here is what you will find in this book—and why I say it's for every woman:

- Chapter 1 tackles ten major myths of menopause, some of which are "absolutes" and others "distortions." The absolutes are false statements that trap women into making bad choices about their health and options to manage menopause symptoms. The distortions have a grain of truth, but lead women toward conclusions about menopause that can be damaging to relationships and harmful to their health.
- Chapter 2 takes you on a trip through a menopausal body—head to toe. In many areas, the narrative explores both the insides, such as the brain, and the outsides, such as the skin.
- Chapter 3 puts the spotlight on hormone therapy. The stories of how hormone therapy got a bad reputation, as well as facts about when it deserves a bad reputation, are punctuated by commentary and insights from experts. Hormone therapy is a divisive topic, particularly when it comes to medical opinions and research about the safety of synthetic hormones versus bioidentical ones.

- Chapter 4 continues the theme of hormones; however, the focus here is on the feel-good hormones of oxytocin, endorphins, serotonin, and dopamine. How can we make more? When do we throw ourselves out of balance by having too much of one and not enough of another? The discussion of feel-good hormones gives insights about the health-related need for intimate relationships as well as how those hormones affect our satisfaction within a relationship.
- Chapter 5 exposes the distinction between libido and sexual motivation, and covers the role of culture in our decisions about intimacy after menopause. Libido is about biology. Sexual motivation is about psychology and emotion. Culture is about socialization—norms, opinions, popular thinking, media, and other profound influences on what we see as options and objectives in a relationship.
- Chapter 6 is the in-depth look at how to address the physical needs a woman in any phase of menopause has when it comes to sexual intimacy. The information in this chapter builds on the discussion of hormone therapy in chapter 3 and looks exclusively at the non-hormone products and techniques that mitigate key symptoms of menopause. Key topics are ending vaginal dryness, cooling hot flashes and night sweats, and overcoming insomnia.
- Chapter 7 features the subject of pleasure—the fact that you deserve it and the process of getting it at all phases of menopause. It offers five steps to achieving greater pleasure in an intimate relationship and includes the in-depth insights of classic experts like William Masters and Virginia Johnson up to modern experts like the instructors of The Welcomed Consensus. A key part of this chapter on viewpoints that engender a "new normal" is the focus on gateway attitudes and emotions: primarily a need to feel safe with your partner and the value of vulnerability in an intimate relationship.
- Chapter 8 offers ways to combine the information about physical needs with a deepened understanding of shifts in viewpoint that can improve intimacy. There are menus of options in this chapter such as sex therapist Jenni Skyler's innovative Cheesecake of Pleasure.
- Chapter 9 explores the force of lifestyle adjustments. Throwing more light on guidance that received just a sentence or two in prior chapters, it emphasizes that menopause as a "change of life" means that women's needs for nutrition, movement, and other lifestyle factors change. The alternative to making these shifts in lifestyle factors is

more severe menopause symptoms, damage to physical and mental health, and increased challenges in maintaining a vibrant intimate life.

• Chapter 10 looks forward. Women's sexual health is not something that has received nearly enough serious research through the years— but that is changing. The sexual dysfunction study led by Dr. Saketh Guntupalli in 2015, with whom I authored the book *Sex and Cancer*, was the first major study of its kind. Some classic studies of hormones, sexual behavior, libido, and more have women's issues as a footnote at best. In contrast, studies now being conducted as well as those on the horizon give us an inkling of new options and revised thinking for menopausal women. This final chapter serves as a bookend to the first in that it approaches the conversation of the "latest and greatest" information through some twenty-first-century myths of menopause. It takes a hopeful look at what upcoming generations of women can expect as they mature.

If this book excites and informs you about showing yourself more respect, then I've succeeded. You should not have to suffer through menopause and/or fret about loss of intimacy because of menopause. You deserve answers and solutions. You deserve pleasure.

Chapter One

Myth versus Reality

Menopause is unnatural. Nearly all animals on the planet can procreate until they die. Humans have done such an exceptional job of sustaining and extending life, however, that the phenomenon of having many non-childbearing years has become common.

Every time a book about menopause is released or an aging celebrity reveals what she's going through, we hear, "How refreshing—we never used to talk about this!" Well, we didn't talk about it because not as many women experienced it. Menopause was a "secret" because it was non-existent or a much briefer period of life for most women.

In 1920, the average life expectancy for a woman in the United States was about fifty-five years. One hundred years later, it's eighty years—a quarter of a century longer to experience menopause and postmenopause. No wonder we're having discussions about it now!

As women began to share anecdotal information about hot flashes, weight gain, and other physical changes associated with an aging body, myths about menopause crept into the conversation. The myths fall into two main categories: absolutes and distortions. Ten common myths could be sorted like this:

Absolutes
Hot flashes are inevitable—and there's not much you can do about them.
You'll gain weight.
Your bones will weaken.

It's okay to leave birth control behind.
Hormone therapy is dangerous.

Distortions
Your sex drive will plummet.
Menopause causes depression.
Menopause is menopause, regardless of whether it is natural or artificial.
Estrogen production stops with menopause.
Start watching for symptoms in your mid-forties.

ABSOLUTES THAT ARE ABSOLUTELY WRONG

Some of the incorrect absolutes that were believed by many women in the twentieth century have been debunked so often that they no longer make the list. They would include "your period just stops one day" and "menopause makes you bad-tempered." There is anecdotal evidence to support both of these myths, of course, but they are far from absolute truths.

In contrast, many women have been told the following five so often that they believe them. As someone I knew who worked in the intelligence community once told me, "If you trust me and I tell you over and over again that the sky is orange, it will eventually look orange to you."

Myth: Hot flashes are inevitable—and there's not much you can do about them.

There is no denying that surveys suggest that eight out of ten menopausal women report that they have had hot flashes, known as night sweats when they occur after bedtime. Look at the data with the flipside perspective: A 2015 study by the University of Pennsylvania confirmed that 20 percent of the women participating had either *no* hot flashes or only mild ones.

Placing the blame solely on the hormonal imbalance occurring with menopause brushes aside the importance of key lifestyle and environmental factors that can affect their occurrence and severity. There are causes and triggers for hot flashes in women besides the drop in estrogen levels, an event that interferes with the body's thermostat.

Two significant triggers are excessive alcohol consumption and smoking cigarettes—but if you overindulge in those two things, hot flashes are probably the least of your health worries. You will also want to avoid the Szechuan sauce and double-shot espresso drinks because spice and caffeine can crank up your temperature. Tight clothing, stress, and dehydration also can contribute to the onset and intensity of hot flashes. Having too much iron in your system has also been documented as a causal factor in hot flashes and night sweats.

Obesity makes the experience worse, too, which is opposite of what people commonly believed until a few years ago. More than one study, including one by the Study of Women's Health Across the Nation concluded that obesity is a risk factor for hot flashes. We used to assume that, as fat cells help produce estrogen, women with more body fat would be protected against severe menopause symptoms. It was a myth that research turned upside down.

Once the correlation between obesity and hot flashes was established, the question was: Does weight loss then reduce the number and severity of the hot flashes? Rebecca Thurston and her team at the Women's Biobehavioral Health Laboratory at the University of Pittsburgh pioneered the work to answer that question. Her 2015 pilot study published in *Menopause* had very promising results; it suggests the answer is "yes."[1]

Quite logically, surgical removal of the ovaries is another trigger. An oophorectomy is a shock to the system, abruptly cutting off the normal flow of estrogen. Women who undergo this procedure can suddenly have severe hot flashes and night sweats. As a corollary, women who have had permanent ovary damage due to chemotherapy or pelvic radiation might also experience the immediate onset of hot flashes.

Nutrient deficiencies can also cause or exacerbate hot flash episodes. The good news here is that correcting a nutritional problem can bring quick relief.

Dr. Carolyn Dean (*Menopause Naturally* and *The Magnesium Miracle*) has extensively researched the effects of magnesium supplementation on menopause as well as collected a wealth of anecdotal evidence through her blog. One of the contributors noticed there seemed to be a match between many of her menopause symptoms—including temperature fluctuations—and symptoms of magnesium deficiency. She decided to increase her intake of magnesium to see what would happen. The magnesium had a rather quick and dramatic impact: "Within three days she began to feel more normal. Her daytime hot flashes had dropped from twenty or so a day to fewer than ten, and they were milder. Her episodes of night sweats fell from more than ten per night to three or less."[2]

There is more good news about relieving symptoms: Certain types and levels of exercise appear to be an effective way to mitigate the number and intensity of hot flashes. Both exercise and hot flashes are thermoregulatory events, but exercise prepares the body to manage the changes much more efficiently.

Here's how exercise and hot flashes are similar:

A hot flash lasting 2-3 minutes can increase cutaneous vasodilation, or surface blood flow, by around 80%; and sweating can be five times more than usual. This is comparable to changes brought about by 30 minutes of moderate-intensity cycling, which tends to raise core body temperature by around 0.4-0.6° Celsius [roughly 33 degrees Fahrenheit].[3]

The main impact of exercise documented in a 2015 study published in *The Journal of Psychology* was the way women who exercised responded to their hot flashes, although it also reduced how often they got them. Primarily, the exercising women were not nearly as sweaty during an episode, and they had more blood flow to the brain. The type of exercises that may help you mitigate symptoms receives more attention in chapter 9 on lifestyle factors.

Myth: You'll gain weight.

Women's Health Network reports that nearly 80 percent of the women who took their Menopause and Perimenopause Quiz last year reported moderate to severe weight gain when their bodies changed.[4] That result could be construed as evidence that the onset of menopause causes weight gain. Anecdotal evidence like that—even an abundance of it—can be deceiving, however.

The common occurrence of weight gain around the time of menopause has led to a belief that it is the primary cause of the numbers rising on the scale. Menopause does cause hormonal changes that make it more likely to gain weight around your middle. But those hormonal changes should not be blamed for weight gain per se.

This is a case of blaming the messenger. Menopause is the messenger delivering the news that you are getting older. In other words, most women should blame their weight gain on aging and the lifestyle changes that often accompany it rather than on menopause.

You can blame *where* the weight goes on hormonal shifts, and that is something explored later in this section. For now, let's stay with the topic of weight gain.

Typically, even athletic women tend to go a little lighter on the exercise regimen as they age. I can speak from experience on this one, having been a competitive athlete for many years and then realizing that my workouts might best be described now as "really taxing . . . for a senior citizen" (senior citizen being defined broadly by AARP as anyone fifty years or older, like Halle Berry, Michelle Pfeiffer, and Madonna). Hit a certain age and everyone in the gym gets concerned seeing an "older woman" do bench presses and deadlifts—and perhaps the most concerned person is me because I fall so short of what I used to do. These are two lifts I excelled in as a competitive powerlifter. Now, I have to admit that my 325-pound deadlift is, well, not that much by 190 pounds.

Muscle mass does not disappear if you do some kind of exercise, but it does diminish with age. And the companion bad news is that fat increases. Loss of muscle mass decreases your body's ability to burn calories. That fact alone can be why a menopausal woman finds it ridiculously hard to maintain a healthy weight. I was throwing around dumbbells for years, but if you were alternating between lifting boxes of supplies at work and carrying toddlers and heavy grocery bags at home, we both worked on building muscle mass that we no longer have.

Without thinking about it (and that's the problem), many women eat as they did during those active years and don't increase their physical activity. Barring some kind of genetic magic, anyone who does that will gain weight.

Speaking of genetics, if there is the potential for magic, there is also the potential for a curse. Genetic factors can affect menopause weight gain. Look at Mom, Grandma, older sisters, aunts, and cousins. It is not likely they will have identical responses to aging, but those who share your lifestyle may give you clues as to your genetic predisposition toward weight gain.

Another incredibly important factor in weight gain is lack of quality sleep. Menopause causes discomfort for many women in the form of sweating and other physiological problems that make a good night's sleep challenging. The results tend to be sporadic, low-quality sleep and snacking when awake to try to get enough energy to get through the day.

Sleep actually reduces your desire for food, whereas sleeplessness triggers the release of ghrelin, also known as the hunger hormone. In a study published in 2016, doctors at the University of Chicago collected abundant evidence that there is a biological interaction between sleep deprivation and weight gain.

Doctors Erin Hanlon and Eve Van Cauter at the University of Chicago noticed:

> Sleep deprivation has effects in the body similar to activation of the endocannabinoid (eCB) system, a key player in the brain's regulation of appetite and energy levels. Perhaps most well-known for being activated by chemicals found in marijuana, the eCB system affects the brain's motivation and reward circuits and can spark a desire for tasty foods.[5]

The people who participated in the study were young—under thirty years—and they were not obese. They adhered to a prescribed diet and allowed either 8.5 hours of sleep or 4.5 hours of sleep for four days in a row. The sleep-deprived participants had eCB levels in the afternoons that were higher and lasted longer than after a full night's quality sleep. Elevation in eCB levels occurred around the same time they reported increases in hunger and appetite.

On the fourth night, the study participants fasted until the following afternoon. At that point, they chose their own meals and snacks for the rest of the day. All of this occurred in a clinical setting so the researchers monitored their choices and intake.

Under both sleep conditions, people consumed about 90 percent of their daily calories at their first meal. But when sleep-deprived, they consumed more and unhealthier snacks between meals. This is when eCB levels were at their highest, suggesting that eCBs were driving hedonic, or pleasurable, eating.

Hanlon's team concluded that seeing junk food after having a good night's sleep does not present the same control challenges as facing junk food after a bad night's sleep: "But if you're sleep deprived, your hedonic drive for certain foods gets stronger, and your ability to resist them may be impaired. . . . Do that again and again, and you pack on the pounds."[6]

If you find yourself in this position of sleep-deprived and hungry, do yourself one favor: Reach for a protein snack instead of a carbohydrate snack. As you age, your requirement for protein increases, so adding a little is probably in your best interests anyway.

Turning to the effects of hormonal shifts on *where* pounds pile up, there is science that says the spare tire relates to changes in levels of estrogen. So a myth of menopause may be weight gain, but it's not a myth that whatever weight you gain will probably go to a place that makes you toss your bikini into the trash.

According to Dr. Pamela Peeke, named one of America's top women physicians by the National Institutes of Health,

> Any woman can get a muffin top. But women are more likely to gain excess belly weight—especially deep inside the belly—as they go through perimenopause and into menopause, when their menstrual cycle ends. That's because as estrogen levels drop, body fat is redistributed from the hips, thighs, and buttocks (where it used to be stored as a fuel reserve for breastfeeding) to the abdomen.[7]

With changes in estrogen levels, your body faces a major challenge: produce more of this hormone to keep your hormones balanced at what your body considered "normal" before menopause. With your ovaries producing less estrogen, your body works at finding other sources. Fat cells produce estrogen, so in an effort to make up for the failure of your ovaries—or in some cases, the total loss of them due to cancer surgery—your body will work to retain fat. It becomes uniquely valuable to your womanhood.

The movie *Sex and the City 2* depicts the sex-obsessed Samantha Jones in an I'll-do-anything-for-estrogen hunt when customs officials in Abu Dhabi confiscate her estrogen supplementation products. She resorts to eating huge quantities of vegetable sources of the hormone, like yams. (More on this during the discussion of bioidenticals in chapter 3.) Someone might have told her just to eat fatty foods, which would ultimately contribute to elevated estrogen levels.

Unfortunately, once fat starts to grow around your middle, you are dealing with the fat equivalent of weeds. The propagation of fat around your waist can seem like a force of nature that cannot be controlled. A number of factors exacerbate the situation, namely stress and the resulting release of cortisol, a steroid hormone that elevates blood sugar.

The second section of this book offers some possibilities for countering the fat problem. In the meantime, here is a tip that won't hurt you
and it may help you a great deal: In counseling obese clients and friends,
and using this guideline myself for a long time, I have found that eliminating wheat, white rice, and refined sugar has a transformative effect
for many people. A resource on this worth reading is William Davis's
Wheat Belly. Davis provides the research behind the recommendation
that weight loss and management is much easier if we eliminate foods
that spike blood sugar.

Myth: Your bones will weaken.

Estrogen has a crucial role in skeletal growth and the stability of bones
in both females and males. Exactly how estrogen deficiency causes
bone loss is not completely understood, however.[8]

We do know this: Menopause is inevitable, but osteoporosis is not.
There is a direct link between a drop in estrogen levels and a decrease in
bone density; however, weight-bearing exercise and nutrition can keep
your bones strong.

Tina and Nancy are the same age; they both graduated from high school
in 1968 so you can figure it out from there. They are both ectomorphs,
meaning they have a delicate build and are very lean. Tina did some fashion modeling in her teens and twenties and developed the habit of eating
very little and never doing strenuous exercise so she wouldn't develop
"manly" muscles. Nancy loved sports and, despite the challenge she had of
putting on muscle—typical for an ectomorph—she was coordinated and
did well at a number of athletic activities. Just after she turned sixty-six,
Tina walked into the open door of her dishwasher and broke her leg. The
year before, she cracked a rib when she hit the soap dish in her shower.
Just after she turned sixty-seven, Nancy summited Mt. Kilimanjaro. At an
elevation of 19,308 feet, it is the highest mountain in Africa.

I know both of these women. One is living proof that a lack of estrogen does nothing more than accelerate the bone-density problems
engendered by a lack of exercise and proper nutrition. The other is
living proof that menopause is not a big deal for your bones if you do
weight-bearing exercises and eat well.

Later in the book, the prevention of osteoporosis receives a lot more
attention, with the roles of hormone therapies, nutrition, and exercise all
coming into the spotlight.

Myth: It's okay to leave birth control behind.

It is not okay, and in fact, perimenopause may be a very good reason to continue birth control pills—perhaps just not the same kind you've probably been taking.

Until you have not had your period for an entire year, you could still get pregnant no matter how many hot flashes you're having. Definitely speak with your doctor about your cycle, or lack thereof, so the two of you are in agreement on when it is safe to stop using birth control or to switch to a low-dose birth control pill for a while. Regular birth control pills contain thirty to fifty micrograms of estrogen, whereas the low-dose pills contain 0.3 to 0.45 micrograms.

Even women who have not been using birth control sometimes go on low-dose birth control pills during perimenopause because the small, additional amount of estrogen can help manage menopausal challenges and fluctuations in hormones. Specific positive effects can be regulating irregular periods and preserving bone strength. The usual cautions apply, however, to women who have a history of blood clots, heart disease, or who either had breast cancer or are genetically predisposed to it.

Chapter 3 takes a much closer look at the potential benefits and hazards of low-dose birth control pills.

Myth: Hormone therapy is dangerous.

As an absolute, this statement is false. Chapter 3 examines in detail how this myth took shape and why it should not be echoed as truth. For some women, hormone therapy provides relief from symptoms, improved health, and an elevated libido. The primary thing to note is that research indicates that starting hormone therapy in the perimenopausal phase of life is the ideal time—if you are an ideal candidate for it.

DISTORTIONS THAT CAN HURT YOUR HEALTH

There is some truth to the myths explored here; however, these statements can veer your thinking toward unhealthy decisions and/or conclusions that will undermine your quality of life.

Myth: Your sex drive will plummet.

The bitter truth is that your desire and satisfaction prior to menopause are key predictors of your desire and satisfaction during and after menopause. The sweet truth is that you can rely on both physical and psychological aids to take both of them up a notch if you want to.

Just as with weight gain, this myth is an example of blaming the messenger. A drop in estrogen and testosterone will affect libido, but to assert that you no longer desire intimacy simply because of menopause means you are denying realities of your relationship that probably pre-dated menopause. Your most powerful sex organ is your brain, which has some "say" as to how much menopause will affect your sex life.

Your brain is also your most powerful sex organ if we take a purely physical look at libido. A complex chain of events begins in the brain, specifically the hypothalamus, that ultimately has an effect on women's ovaries (and men's testicles), leading to the production of testosterone. The hypothalamus is a tiny region at the base of the brain that has a vital role in releasing hormones, regulating body temperature, maintaining daily psychological cycles, controlling appetite, managing sexual responses, and regulating emotional responses.[9]

The hormone fueling sex drive is testosterone—an androgen, and the so-called male hormone. While production of it does decrease with age, the menopause-related decrease in estrogen might give testosterone more dominance in your biochemistry. That appears to be the reason why some women experience increased libido during menopause.

Now we get to the upward spiral of testosterone production. When the desire to have more sex leads to having more sex, it appears that a woman's testosterone levels increase. Several studies have looked at changes in the endocrine system evoked by orgasmic events and the results indicate that more begets more.[10]

Testosterone production peaks in a woman's twenties. By the time menopause occurs, the level is half of what it was then. Even after the ovaries stop delivering estrogen to the body, they still make testosterone, a small amount of which is also produced by the adrenal glands. Even with testosterone levels dropping in both men and women as they age, the fuel tank is not empty. Staying physically active, particularly including resistance training, can increase the amount of testosterone circulating in your system.

Chapter 3 delves more deeply into the roles of the key hormones of estrogen, progesterone, and testosterone, and how replenishing the supplies can have a physical effect on libido. Chapter 4 adds to that discussion with a look at how to generate the "happy hormones" that enhance your satisfaction during and after intimate encounters.

Myth: Menopause causes depression.

Shifts in hormones can certainly create mood swings, but as of this writing, there is no credible study that makes menopause a causal factor in depression. That does not mean that menopause is off the hook as a legitimate reason to feel down and anxious, however. There are a number of reasons why a woman might feel depressed during menopause, and we should never negate them. In dealing with daily disruptions of symptoms such as hot flashes a dozen times a day—while they conduct meetings and attend social events—women in menopause can get emotionally fatigued and depressed. And for women who still want children and find themselves thrust into menopause due to disease or treatment for a disease, the sense of loss could have a profound impact on their mental health.

Women experiencing ongoing moderate to severe symptoms are at risk for depression. That is not the same as asserting that menopause causes depression, but it can create a context for it. Each woman has the good, the bad, and the ugly of menopause—and each experience and story is different for each woman.

Rooting the discussion in physiological reasons for depression during menopause, we can look at how testosterone deficiency and estrogen deprivation can affect a menopausal woman's mental state and have her arrive at the conclusion that she is depressed.

Having just read the above description of how testosterone affects libido, consider that it is an essential part of your biochemistry and a deficiency in it will affect mood. To summarize one outcome of studies: "Because testosterone is a hormone, symptoms of deficiency resemble symptoms of depression and other mood disorders. In fact, certain experts argue that misdiagnosis and lack of treatment are common for these reasons."[11]

Estrogen also has a function in regulating moods. It affects parts of the brain that determine how we respond emotionally to events. Among other things, estrogen plays a role in:

• Increasing serotonin, and the propagation of serotonin receptors in the brain.
• Modifying the production and the effects of endorphins, which are also known as "feel-good" chemicals in the brain.
• Protecting nerves from damage, and possibly stimulating nerve growth.[12]

When you are perimenopausal, estrogen levels fluctuate in an unpredictable way. The up and down is enough to make most women feel depressed, at least occasionally. The above reference to the value of taking a low-dose birth control pill relates directly to mitigating this symptom of perimenopause.

During menopause, when estrogen levels plummet, there are a few choices if you feel depressed, and they include taking estrogen supplements, taking antidepressants (which may have a negative impact on your libido), and waiting it out. After menopause, women's rates of depression seem to fall.

Please note well: **Menopause may be a life-changing event that triggers awareness of clinical depression.** Anyone who can say, "I'm depressed" would benefit from sharing that with a licensed therapist and her regular doctor.

Myth: Menopause is menopause, regardless of whether it is natural or artificial.

Natural menopause has three stages: perimenopause, menopause, and postmenopause, or before, during, and after. Artificial menopause has only the latter two.

In many cases, a woman facing the possibility of surgical menopause has very little—or no—time to prepare psychologically, physically, or emotionally. There is a serious, perhaps life-and-death, need to act quickly and radically.

At the age of forty-two years, wellness coach and lifelong athlete Lori Ann King went to the doctor after having some cramping and digestive issues. Due to a history of colon cancer in her family, she had been going for regular screenings and followed up with her gastroenterologist. The doctor found nothing irregular, but the symptoms continued, so she recommended a magnetic resonance imaging and computed tomography scan. Those tests revealed an ovarian cyst and what was simply called a "mass near your uterus." She ultimately learned that there was a 90 percent chance that the "mass"—a terrifying term in any diagnostic situation—was actually a fibroid. Going on the diagnosis of "mass," however, she and her husband decided to get it removed and take a wait-and-see approach with the cyst. The mass was indeed a fibroid so phase one of the experience let King breathe a sigh of relief.

The initial surgery took place just before the winter holidays, and by January, she felt strong enough to attend a wellness convention. Ironically, she soon became as unwell as she'd ever been. She collapsed and was carted off to a nearby hospital in an ambulance.

In the coming weeks, the cyst continued to grow and King and her husband decided it would be best to have it removed rather than risk having it burst. The probable outcome was that she would be left one ovary and return to her normal active life quickly. The worst-case scenario—a total hysterectomy—seemed highly unlikely. That would only occur if the endometriosis had spread throughout her reproductive organs. No one gave her the "big book of answers" on what she might face with the worst-case scenario.

King woke up and learned that she no longer had ovaries, a uterus, fallopian tubes, or a cervix. She didn't just have a total hysterectomy; she had a total hysterectomy with a bilateral salpingo-oophorectomy. Lori Ann King had been dumped on Planet Menopause.

> All of a sudden we were talking about hormone therapy, where do we go from here, and how long is this healing going to take. I was feeling unprepared and like I had no control over my emotions. I felt out of focus, scared, and confused. I also had to go into a quick acceptance, "Okay, I knew this was a possibility. I gave my doctor and my husband permission to make this decision. It was the worst-case scenario. Now what?"[13]

King found that the time frame and intensity of her menopause symptoms differed markedly from those of women, including her sister, who were going through a natural menopause. There was nothing gradual about the process with periods going from steady to sporadic to non-existent. No surfacing of symptoms over time. Instead, at the age of forty-three years, despite starting bioidentical hormone therapy within a week of her surgery, she suddenly had the whole menu of menopausal unpleasantries: hot flashes, night sweats, insomnia, fatigue, low libido, and anxiety.

In addition to surgery, chemotherapy and pelvic radiation are among the other potential causes of irreversible damage to the ovaries that can abruptly stop their functioning. With all of these treatments, there is an immediate deficit in the body's supply of estrogen, progesterone, and testosterone.

Due to her experience as an athlete and wellness coach, King is very body aware. She also has experience with both mainstream and complementary approaches to mitigating menopause systems and offers a wealth of them in her book *Come Back Strong: Balanced Wellness after Surgical Menopause.*

Her path to toning down some terrible symptoms was a long one. After sixteen months of using a bioidentical topical therapy, she was still battling symptoms, including weight gain. Her doctor and her friends suggested that she try life without hormone therapy and happily assured her that the extra weight would disappear. Not only did her weight problem continue after weaning herself from the hormone cream, but she also soon realized that not having the hormones made hot flashes and night sweats an even more acute presence in her life. And to exacerbate the unpleasantness, in the five months without any hormone therapy, she also experienced vaginal atrophy.

That's when she went running back to her doctor and went back on hormone therapy.

That alone could not salvage her quality of life, however.

Ultimately, King built a program for herself that included hormones, as well as treatments such as acupuncture and chiropractic. And the physical training went up a notch. As soon as she had been cleared for it by her doctor, she went back to cycling, yoga, and weight training, but as time (and symptoms) went on, she grew even more committed to lifestyle changes that would help her feel normal again.

> Acupuncture was a hugely important modality for me. I had started acupuncture before my hysterectomy and then continued. My acupuncturist always treated me as a whole person. I would go to her with symptoms and she would ask me all sorts of different questions. To an Eastern

medicine practitioner, every detail matters. Whereas I wouldn't connect the dots in my head, she would connect the dots in hers to get a more complete picture of how my symptoms might be interrelated.[14]

King succeeded in regaining her quality of life. A piece of her early journey into reconnecting with her husband is included in chapter 6. It's an exuberant reminder that, even in the midst of horrific symptoms, it is possible to use the tools at hand, including your attitude, to manage menopause.

Myth: Estrogen production stops with menopause.

This is not true, but because the slow-down of estrogen production can be dramatic, it is often embraced as true. With the ovaries no longer manufacturing estrogen, the assumption is that the supply dries up. The ovaries and the adrenal glands, which are located on top of the kidneys, do continue to produce a hormone called androstenedione, which is converted into estrogen. Fat cells also contribute to estrogen production.

Making the assumption that there is zero estrogen in your body at menopause can drive you to some bad health decisions. Your body is still making estrogen (and testosterone), and a healthful plan of attack is to ascertain if you want to do something to supplement your body's "production facilities." If so, the next discussion to have with your physician is what that course of action is.

Myth: Start watching for symptoms in your mid-forties.

With the average age of the onset of menopause established at about fifty-one years,[15] it would seem logical to look for signs of perimenopause in your mid-forties. However, perimenopause "is an ill-defined time period that surrounds the final years of a woman's reproductive life,"[16] according to an in-depth 2016 study published in the *Journal of Women's Health*. The onset of perimenopause can occur in a woman's thirties.

Ignoring symptoms, or perhaps worse yet, assuming that all body changes are symptoms of menopause, can get you into trouble.

If you ignore symptoms, you could miss the opportunity to begin hormone therapy when it might be a truly healthful, beneficial choice. The timing of hormone therapy is discussed in much greater depth in chapter 3.

And then there is the story of Cherie, who watched for symptoms and neglected to see other signs. She was forty-two years old and a physician's assistant at a regional clinic. Cherie had irregular periods and thought nothing of it because she thought she was going into a perimenopausal phase. Unfortunately, some of the irregular bleeding— which she never discussed with her gynecologist—was due to a tumor in her uterus. By the time she sought the proper medical attention, she was diagnosed with stage III endometrial cancer. The happy news is that she had aggressive treatment and is fine. The cautionary tale is that every woman needs to pay attention to changes in her cycles and perceived changes in her reproductive organs no matter how old she is. Do not let myths cloud your judgment about the realities of your body and what it needs to stay healthy.

Chapter Two

Menopause Head to Toes

Having dispelled a few prime menopause myths, we can now look at what really is going on, or might be going on, all over your body. The grain of truth in many of the myths is rooted in a superficial understanding of what happens inside and outside the body with the onset of menopause. This chapter will help you get to know more about your hormones, organs, muscles, and bones, and how they evolve as you mature.

Familiarity with the physical changes that occur during the perimenopausal and menopausal phases of life leads to an understanding of expected effects, as well as surprising effects such as allergies, body odor, and brittle nails. It may be socially acceptable to grumble occasionally about hot flashes, but if a menopausal woman brings up her difficulty in finding an effective deodorant, she might be dismissed as a chronic complainer.

These are real symptoms, however, that can not only affect daily life, but also add to the list of reasons why a mature woman has physical and psychological challenges in her sex life.

HEAD

The head includes the brain, of course, the source of the biochemical changes occurring as part of menopause. The cosmetic, external changes that occur in the head and neck are daily reminders of those unstoppable internal changes. Once we explore what biochemical stops and starts are occurring in the brain during the menopause transition, we have the foundation for understanding many of the other conditions and effects associated with menopause. The brain is also a pleasure machine and remains one during and after menopause.

THE BRAIN

Role in Menopause

Women going through menopause crave information about symptoms and how to relieve them, and the internet is full of tips and insights. It is much harder to come across accessible explanations of the mechanics of changes in the brain before, during, and after menopause.

We talk a great deal about hot flashes, vaginal dryness, and sleeplessness in this book; however, the vague explanation of why they occur—hormone fluctuations—doesn't really explain what is happening biochemically. The answer lies in the brain.

A stripped-down description of the process is that the brain sends signals to the ovaries to release an egg once a month from the onset of puberty and then won't shut up when the ovaries can no longer perform on schedule. Release of the egg corresponds to estrogen production. The unrelenting signals start a chain reaction resulting in certain menopausal symptoms as the ovaries attempt to "do their job" and produce estrogen.

As far as we know now, a woman's ovaries contain all the egg cells she will ever have when she is born. The estimate is in the millions, with thousands dying every month; by the time a female reaches puberty, she ends up with about four hundred thousand. The egg cells are contained in tiny, fluid-filled pockets called follicles. When the egg supply diminishes to about one thousand, a woman is perimenopausal. The hypothalamus and pituitary gland are not aware of this short supply, however, so they continue to do what they had done every month of every year since the woman hit puberty. The hypothalamus sends a hormone called gonadotropin-releasing hormone to the pituitary gland and it responds by releasing follicle-stimulating hormone to get the ovary to release a follicle.

These parts of the brain, therefore, are essentially saying, "Hello, down there! We would like you to make more estrogen . . . and we will keep sending you this annoying message until you respond!"

As explained briefly in chapter 1, one function of the hypothalamus is to regulate body temperature. With it becoming overactive in releasing gonadotropin-releasing hormone, there is a strong possibility that the body will heat up. Fluctuations in estrogen levels are associated with many of the other symptoms described in this chapter.

Role in Orgasm

Given the emphasis of this book on intimacy during and after menopause, a discussion of the brain would be incomplete without referencing how it participates in sexual pleasure at all phases of life. A team of researchers led by Emmanuele A. Jannini, a well-known researcher in sexual medicine, elegantly described the brain's involvement in the opening of their paper "Peripheral and Central Neural Bases of Orgasm":

> In the central nervous system during orgasm, essentially all of the major brain systems are activated, including the brainstem, limbic system, cerebellum, and cortex. In a symphony of integration, these peripheral and central systems mediate the sensory, cognitive, autonomic, and motor events of orgasm.[1]

Among the events that occur is the release of dopamine, a neurotransmitter that could be described as your body's "reward chemical." Dopamine neurons are activated when something enjoyable occurs, like orgasm or a great dessert. Production of it, and more detail about its value to your sex life, is covered in chapter 4 on the "feel good hormones." In short, your brain is a full and vital participant in anything pleasurable that happens in the body no matter how old you are.

Cognitive Issues and Menopause

Contrary to popular belief, hormone fluctuations are not *directly* responsible for every annoying thing that happens during menopause. Studies testing the effect of hormone changes on cognitive ability have been inconclusive, but those that seemed to establish a link led to an uptick in hormone replacement therapy. Other studies concluded the opposite: that is, hormone therapy (HT) made the problem worse. The latest thinking is that oscillations in estrogen levels do not cause issues with fuzziness or memory lapses: They cause other issues that ultimately contribute to cognitive difficulties and once those issues are addressed, the cognitive impairment should disappear.

Estrogen is an important part of the biochemistry affecting mood and sleep, and it is actually impaired sleep and inconsistent moods that trigger memory and other cognitive issues, not the loss of estrogen per se.[2] One study on the influence of estrogen on cognitive changes after menopause opened with this definitive statement: "The natural menopause is not associated with substantial cognitive change."[3] Other studies affirm this conclusion.[4]

The situation seems to be different for women who have undergone surgical menopause. The abrupt cessation of estrogen production appears to be linked to some temporary cognitive impairment, particularly memory loss; unfortunately, clinical evidence does not support the theory that HT would help.[5]

Regardless of whether aging or disease-related therapies have caused menopause, addressing the sleeplessness and stress in your life appears to be the primary action to alleviate symptoms such as memory loss, lack of ability to concentrate, and tension headaches.

Elevated and depressed levels of hormones can also cause menopausal headaches. Estrogen causes blood vessels to dilate, with progesterone having the opposite effect. Fluctuations in both of them could cause a throbbing headache as blood vessels are forced to expand and constrict.

THE HEAD AND NECK

Hair Loss

In interviewing countless cancer patients for *Sex and Cancer*, which I wrote with Saketh Guntupalli, I learned how devastated women were at the loss of their hair. I lost mine, too, so this was a personal message. A gynecologic oncologist, Dr. Guntupalli also noted that the majority of his patients who lost their hair due to chemotherapy expressed everything from disappointment to profound anxiety at the loss of a key symbol of their style, femininity, and sexuality.

Unfortunately, hair loss to some degree is also a symptom of peri-menopause. Unlike post-chemo trauma, you won't slide your fingers through your hair and come up with a clump, but you may notice thinning. Levels of estrogen and testosterone both drop during menopause and they are both important to the quality and quantity of hair on your head. Thank estrogen for fast-growing, thick, healthy hair. Thank testosterone for preventing hair loss. And go ahead: Curse menopause for taking an abundant supply of each away from you.

Wrinkly Skin

Collagen production decreases as well. Your skin has less elasticity and doesn't seem as plump. Wrinkles show up. You listen to ads for expensive miracle serums and calculate in your mind how many venti soy lattes you have to give up in order to afford them. On the positive side, if you did give up those lattes (and therefore the caffeine and sugar) and put that money into gathering and ingesting fruits and vegetables of every color imaginable (that is, antioxidant sources), your new diet would help strengthen your skin, as would ensuring you have enough protein in your diet. In addition to using those serums, there is a good chance you could look younger, or at least pull the plug on the biological clock for a while. If you add vigorous exercise to the mix, you have an effective way of combating the skin-aging effects of menopause. Getting your heart rate up through lifting weights, yoga, jogging, cycling, or walking the golf course will boost circulation, which slows with age.

Although the external changes may be unstoppable, women who are good candidates for HT have the opportunity to slow those changes down and retain some of the cosmetic plusses of their younger days. There are also non-hormonal products, some of which were referenced previously, that can nourish the mature skin and scalp in ways that make a visible difference.

Mouth Problems

A surprising number of women entering menopause—estimated to be up to 40 percent[6]—experience a burning sensation in the mouth. Burning mouth syndrome has been the subject of a number of medical papers; however, one of particular interest to this discussion was published in the Polish journal devoted to menopause research.

The research team from Poznan University of Medical Sciences noted in their abstract:

> The hypothesis concerning the role of hormonal changes in the development of BMS [burning mouth syndrome] seems to be confirmed by a high incidence of this condition in perimenopausal women. Up to now, due to an unclear etiology of the disease, the treatment is very often ineffective and mainly symptomatic, which may exacerbate patients' anxiety and discomfort.[7]

By the end of the paper, the discussion of treatment held some promise. The team noted that many women with the condition had reduced pain after HT. Keep in mind that the focus was on perimenopausal women; the potential advantages of beginning HT early were noted previously and are explored in more detail in chapter 3.

Gum problems and dry mouth might also surface at the onset of menopause. Some of the problems can be attributed to the aging process; men experience things like gum tissue recession, too. But estrogen does affect oral tissues, so menopause is a time to take extra steps to maintain oral health.

ARMS AND HANDS

A tingling sensation and/or numbness are relatively uncommon symptoms of menopause, but since estrogen affects the central nervous system, they are possible. Generally, the pins-and-needles feeling and/or numbness—called paresthesia—affects the arms and hands and/or legs and feet, but it could affect the entire body. Variations of paresthesia could be any of the following:

- Tingling
- Numbness
- Burning
- Crawly feeling
- Hypersensitivity

By themselves, if the symptoms come and go during menopause, just report them as part of your normal conversation with your doctor. But if they are combined with pain, spasms, weakness or paralysis, vision changes, an injury, difficulties with speech or walking, fainting, or loss of sensation on one side of the body, the recommendation is that you seek medical attention.[8] The latter list of issues could be a sign that something other than menopause is causing the tingling and/or numbness.

Your manicurist may notice another symptom of menopause before you do: brittle nails. Along with that might be changes in the color, surface ridges, and slower nail growth. Because nail issues are primarily cosmetic, this symptom generally doesn't appear on lists of indicators or annoyances of menopause. Yes, it is one more sign that your hormones are oscillating. It can also signal that you are not getting a sufficient amount of protein in your diet.

Joint issues in the arms and hands are also a problem caused by a reduction in estrogen production. The discussion of joint pain is in the section on hips and legs.

BREASTS

Breasts tend to swell up just before a woman's period because the hormonal changes cause a fluid buildup. Similarly, fluctuations in hormone levels with the onset of perimenopause can cause swelling, tenderness, and even pain. Some women experience extreme pain in their nipples, to the point where they'd rather be nudists because the touch of clothing is a horrible feeling.

Unfortunately, because the menstrual cycle is no longer regular in perimenopause, the discomfort becomes unpredictable. For many women, a sports bra would be more comfortable than a regular dress model because of the way it conforms to the body. A bra made of cotton with just a small percentage of spandex and no underwire should provide support and be breathable enough to be tolerable even during hot flashes.

And now the reason why women of a certain age really need to do pushups if they are physically able to do so: With menopause, glandular tissue shrinks because we no longer need the ability to produce milk. The breasts become fattier at the same time they lose density, so they sag. If you hate pushups or should not do them because you have issues with your pelvic floor or have joint issues, free weights or machines are an option for targeting the area. You could also enjoy the many types of activities that give your upper body a workout like golf, tennis, or swimming.

A scary symptom of menopause that some women experience is lumps in the breast. **They must be checked by your physician** promptly, even though they might just be cysts. The presence of cysts does not mean you are cancer prone, by the way. These lumps might disappear after menopause, or they might remain, particularly if you are using HT to replenish your estrogen supply. The story of Joan, which is among those in chapter 3, includes her experience of breast lumps and repeated mammograms throughout the time she was on HT.

ABDOMEN

We will define abdomen here as the area internally and externally that is below the breasts and above the pelvis. The discussion of the pelvic area will include the reproductive organs, but in this section, we'll look at everything else that belongs to this middle ground.

Symptoms commonly attributed to perimenopause and menopause include constipation and diarrhea, although it doesn't appear to be the shift in hormone levels that cause them. A 2018 study published in the journal *Menopause* concluded that "key reproductive hormones do not play a significant role in constipation or diarrhea severity in the MT [menopause transition]. In contrast, stress perception, tension, anxiety, and cortisol do." In other words, it's the byproducts of hormone shifts that cause the symptoms, but they are experienced enough to be commonly reported as symptoms of perimenopause and menopause.[9]

Urinary incontinence is a common problem for menopausal women, with causes potentially being several interrelated effects of hormone shifts. This is a symptom to pay attention to because it does not tend to go away as you move out of the main menopausal years—it often gets worse. As you age, this problem could not only become increasingly disruptive to your sleep, social life, and career obligations, but also to your love life.

Main reasons for urinary incontinence come down to these:

• During menopause, the pelvic floor muscles tend to weaken. One possible result is less bladder control and more frequent urination.

- A pelvic organ prolapse is a slipping forward or sagging downward of organs against the pelvic floor. The organs in this area include your bladder, uterus, vagina, small bowel, and rectum. A prolapse strains your pelvic floor to the point where incontinence results.
- The base of your bladder can lose elasticity. You may have been someone who could sit through a five-hour meeting before, but with menopause, you may lose the elasticity that allowed that. Your bladder could then get irritated as it fills, causing a feeling you have to go to the bathroom more often.
- With menopause, your body is more susceptible to incontinence because there isn't enough estrogen to help keep the tissues around your bladder resilient.
- Since your pelvic floor muscles support much of your body weight, any excess weight strains these muscles; they are less able to support your bladder as they should. The result is called stress incontinence.

Depending on the primary reason for the incontinence, the solution could be different from person to person. Pelvic floor therapies, HT, surgery, and other solutions receive attention later in this book as we explore the many ways to improve intimate contact through symptom mitigation. To give you a preview, a large study confirmed that non-surgical treatment of stress incontinence led to improved sexual function for a preponderance of women in the study.

Bloating is another abdominal symptom. The water retention and/or buildup of intestinal gas causing the bloating can both be side effects of fluctuating estrogen levels. Just as women tend to retain more water right before their period when estrogen levels rise, when they go up and down during perimenopause, the bloating can come and go. Estrogen also impacts production of bile, the alkaline fluid that aids digestion of fats. When the body does not digest fats properly, bloating is one likely result. Finally, bloating can also result from HT.

PELVIC AREA

Just as we did with the head, we need to look both inside and outside with the pelvic area. In this case, the "brain" is the reproductive system we can't see, yet it is effecting massive changes throughout the body. Outside, there are critical pleasure areas, that is, everything exterior to the vaginal opening. The drama associated with menopause and loss of intimacy occurs both inside and outside.

Over the course of decades, the typical female body kicks out an egg from the ovary every month until she runs out. She is left with no more eggs and just a trickle of estrogen along with some testosterone.

Warnings about decreases in sensation and pleasure come with just about every book and article covering symptoms of menopause. By this time, the reasons are probably well known to you: low estrogen triggers vaginal atrophy and dryness, and with age comes a diminished blood supply to the clitoris and lower vagina.

All of this should be followed by a "*however . . .*" However, while these changes do occur, women who remain sexually active, either through pleasing themselves or enjoying intimate relations with a partner, essentially overcome the ravages of aging. The opposite is true, too. It is a use it or lose it challenge.

The vagina gets a great deal of attention in chapter 6, so in this summary, we will say simply that this center of pleasure will steadily decline into a source of discomfort or even pain if a perimenopausal or menopausal woman fails to be proactive in countering symptoms. What may come as a surprise is that it is also true for the clitoris. Even with its spectacular eight thousand nerve endings in the glans, if it is not stimulated, the clitoris can lose its ability to function.

With all of the "bad" news in this chapter about the deleterious effects of low estrogen levels, let's focus for a moment on a body part that can remain fully functional and healthy with very little effort throughout menopause and beyond.

The clitoris is an astonishing organ that does not have to become as old as the rest of you—and it is an organ that is more complicated than most people think. It begins as a visible spot and then becomes hidden as it loops into the body. Most of us grow up thinking it's just the bulb that is part of the vulva. Instead, it's a multi-faceted structure and, as such, is more appropriately called the "clitoral complex." Externally, it consists of[10]:

- the glans, or the small circular mass that is the visible part of the clitoral complex;

- the prepuce, also commonly called "the hood," which is the skin likened to the penile foreskin; and
- the frenulum, a posterior fold.

Internally, where most of the erectile tissue is, it consists of[11]:

- the body—a pair of corpus cavernosum—not a spell uttered by Hermione Granger in *Harry Potter*, but rather two masses of erectile tissue;
- the bulbs, also called the clitoral vestibules; and
- two crura, which are two pieces of erectile tissue that surround the urethra.

The clitoris divides twice as it weaves through the body. The first time it bifurcates, it goes off in the direction of the hip and, during arousal, becomes larger and longer. It continues around and goes along the vaginal opening. Depending on how far it loops around can affect a woman's sensations in that area.

Incidentally, the internal structure of the clitoris went unstudied until the 1990s when researchers began using magnetic resonance imaging to document the structures. And we didn't know how the entire clitoris behaved while aroused until 2009 when ultrasound studies confirmed what happened with the inside portion of the clitoral complex.

Alas it wasn't until as recent as 2009, French researchers Dr. Odile Buisson and Dr. Pierre Foldès gave the medical world its first complete 3-D sonography of the stimulated clitoris. They did this work for three years without any proper funding. Thanks to them, we now understand how the erectile tissue of the clitoris engorges and surrounds the vagina—a complete breakthrough that explains how what we once considered to be a vaginal orgasm is actually an internal clitoral orgasm.[12]

Sensual rubbing can cause the internal clitoris to become erect; glans, bulbs, and crura all get stimulated from the outside. The corpus cavernosum, the erectile tissue encompassing the vagina, gets stimulated from the inside.

This internal stimulation of the clitoral complex is the key to the elusive Gräfenberg spot, or G spot, once thought to be a distinct anatomical structure. Dr. Beverly Whipple (*The G Spot*) is the researcher who identified the G spot as part of her investigation into female urinary incontinence. We now know that stimulating the spot is actually a clitoral arousal.

Along with all the happy news that sexual arousal and satisfaction are achievable during and after menopause, there is the reality that more effort generally needs to be invested in the process. Whipple explains:

> Menopausal women have less erotic response to stimulation—vulva, clitoris, breasts, and nipples—and more difficulty focusing on tactile sensations that previously created a state of sexual arousal.[13]

The anatomical ability to experience extreme pleasure, therefore, remains throughout and after menopause, but arousal is not likely to happen with the same ease it once did. Celebrate the fact that you can still experience it as long as you want to, and then, through self-stimulation and intimate encounters with your partner, stay in practice.

HIPS AND LEGS

Even without the complication of menopause, women are more likely to have joint pain than men. This is due in part to our being more flexible; the additional range of motion puts women at greater risk for developing joint pain. Add a decrease in estrogen and women are even more susceptible to joint pain because estrogen appears to affect the condition of cartilage, the flexible tissues that provide cushioning at the joints.[14]

The reasoning behind putting this discussion in a section on the lower body is that weight gain can profoundly affect joint pain in the hips and knees. Combining a loss of estrogen with obesity puts a woman at high risk for joint pain in these areas. At first, the pain may be what's commonly called "menopausal arthritis," and it might diminish over time. But the extra weight and less resilient cartilage are a double whammy that could lead to lifelong aches. At the first sign of joint pain, talk to a physical therapist and/or your doctor about lifestyle changes that can alleviate it or even eliminate it.

FEET AND TOES

A UK-based forum called Mumsnet has active discussions on a number of topics of interest to parents, particularly women. The menopause discussion board quickly drew thirty-nine posts when one fifty-one-year-old member asked if her sore feet and ankles could be due to menopause. Other women roughly her age shared the symptoms, with one fifty-three-year-old chiming in:

> I had sore and stiff ankles for months. I've only just realised, reading your thread, that I no longer have them!
>
> Since starting HRT [hormone replacement therapy], 2 months ago, that, along with hot flushes, insomnia, low moods, irritability, zero libido, itching and thinking everyone I live and work with, or indeed come across, is an idiot; has gone! Vanished!![15]

The "miracle cure" this woman experienced may relate to the fact that fluctuations in estrogen levels, and the ultimate decline, can cause fluid retention. Swollen, sore feet and ankles are one possible result. In addition, any problems in that area that already existed, such as bunions and corns, can get much worse. HT could have easily alleviated the problem of swelling.

Some women have foot discomfort mostly at night; they feel as though their feet are on fire. The stress of menopause can lead to depletion of B vitamins, so this could be one cause. Another, which should be addressed by your doctor, is high blood pressure.

Aging alone brings on foot problems. Just as you are gaining fat around the middle from menopause, your feet are losing the fat they need to provide cushioning. You may need a few pairs of good insoles to ensure you're not walking on skin and bones.

Women who struggle with weight gain during menopause may also find themselves aching for shoes that are well-cushioned, as well as a bit larger than before. The added pressure from weight gain on the foot's twenty-six bones, thirty-three joints, and more than 120 muscles, ligaments, tendons, and nerves can make menopause even more uncomfortable than it is with symptoms directly caused by estrogen loss.

After three months of doing personal training with a short fifty-two-year-old woman who weighed two hundred pounds, we got her down to 165 and she declared victory. At her "graduation" ceremony in the gym, I told her to close her eyes and stand with her feet slightly apart and her knees slightly bent. I said, "I'm going to give you something very heavy to hold, so be prepared." I handed her a thirty-five-pound dumbbell and said, "Open your eyes." She looked down at the dumbbell and dropped it on the floor. "That's heavy! It made my feet hurt!"

"That's what you were carrying around for ten years," I told her. Your feet will speak to you when you are carrying excess weight—and you won't like what they say.

THE WHOLE BODY

Two symptoms of menopause generally receive little attention because they don't tend to be as dramatic as raging hot flashes. They are allergies and body odor.

Allergies occur when your immune system is triggered by something like pollen, dust, food, or any number of environmental ingested substances. In menopause, just as in any other phase of life when hormone levels are changing, sensitivity to irritating substances can increase. For some women, brand new allergies surface during menopause.

In terms of your intimate life, one of the most annoying manifestations of an allergy may be an itchy rash or hives. Other issues, like irritated eyes and sneezing, might be easily addressed by an antihistamine. Skin rashes, however, can persist as an irritating and even ugly reminder that you are going through big changes.

The first course of action is to attempt to remove the source of the irritation. And even if you have no food allergies, it would be wise to remove foods from your diet that cause inflammation in the body. Some of the major offenders are processed meats, sodas, fatty foods, wheat products (bread, cake, and so on), and many snack foods like chips and pretzels.

For some women, a combination of the extra sweating and stress caused by hormonal shifts causes changes in body odor. In addition to handling this in the usual ways, consider adding more magnesium to your diet. There do not appear to be any scientific studies about the effects of magnesium on body odor; however, there is scientific speculation and anecdotal evidence. The original source of the science is Pierre Delbet, a French surgeon who discovered benefits of magnesium chloride for the wounded in World War I. He used it topically to cleanse wounds because it did not damage tissues the way antiseptics did. After that, he found it could be taken orally to improve other conditions, such as an imbalance in intestinal bacteria that might cause foul body odor.[16]

Five symptoms seem to dominate discussions of menopause, and it's probably because they cause so many women a great deal of anxiety: hot flashes/night sweats, weight gain, osteoporosis, loss of libido, and mood swings. Chapter 1 introduced all of them, citing causes and, in some cases, hinting at solutions.

The next chapter delves deeply into one category of solutions that is at the heart of controversy in the medical community: HT. Medical professionals arguing in favor of it say women who are good candidates can be confident using it to alleviate the symptoms like hot flashes that affect the whole body. Those arguing against it assert that it is not worth the risk, not as effective as other therapies, or undesirable because it interferes with nature. As we explore the arguments, we'll continue looking at why symptoms occur and whether they can—and should—be stopped by HT.

Non-hormonal therapies dominate later chapters and address alternatives to HT that have science, or at least substantial anecdotal evidence, to indicate they are useful in restoring health and intimate life during and after menopause.

Chapter Three

Pros and Cons of Hormone Therapy

A tsunami of misinformation about the effects of hormone replacement therapy has frightened women since the dawn of this century. To be correct, however, let's abandon the term hormone replacement therapy in favor of just hormone therapy (HT), as the HT is not designed to replace what had been the amounts the body previously produced, but rather to relieve symptoms associated with menopause and prevent any ill effects caused by reduced estrogen in the body. If anything, it might better be called hormone supplement therapy, rather than hormone replacement therapy.

Yes, there can be dangers in having HT, whether it involves synthetic hormones or bioidentical hormones, both of which are explained here. Not every woman faces the dangers, however. In fact, many women will feel younger, stronger, healthier, and be more sexually active with HT.

This chapter explores what we know about risk factors as well as who might be a great candidate for one of the many therapies approved for use in the United States, Europe, and/or other countries.

HORMONE THERAPY'S IMAGE PROBLEM

The primary genesis of widespread fear about HT in the United States was the Women's Health Initiative (WHI) study, which was planned as an 8.5-year effort and aborted just after the five-year mark due to serious health problems encountered by some participants. That news broke in 2002:

> A large federal study of hormone replacement therapy in postmenopausal women was abruptly halted, researchers say, because the drugs caused a slight but significant increase in the risk of invasive breast cancer.[1]

At the time this story made headlines, an estimated sixteen million women in the United States were taking hormones to counter the natural loss of estrogen due to menopause, according to the Stanford Prevention Research Center of the Stanford University School of Medicine. After the WHI study results hit the news, use of HT plummeted 64 percent among women sixty years or older, 60 percent among women between fifty and fifty-nine years, and 59 percent among women younger than fifty years.[2] In the United Kingdom, where the Million Women Study published in 2003 collected similar results through a survey, there was an overall decline of 66 percent.[3] The HT use-rate remained at that low level for the remainder of the decade, in part because of additional negative reports that followed in the years to come.

> The new report on dementia, being published today in the *Journal of the American Medical Association*, is one more piece of bad news about hormone therapy. Indeed, it is the latest in a string of studies showing that purported benefits do not exist and that the hormones actually raise the risk of several serious diseases, including some they were thought to prevent.[4]

The *New York Times* and other distinguished news sources delivered the bad news without realizing that the study on HT that prompted it had been the victim of flawed analysis and interpretation. The sensational reporting was grossly misleading and contributed to fears about HT that persist to this day. The alarming articles gave rise to a belief about the dangers of HT that was as bizarre as the belief that lemmings make suicidal plunges off cliffs during migration. We can chide Disney for the latter—lemmings were involuntarily hurled into the Arctic Sea for the film *White Wilderness*—and we can chastise the WHI for the former.

Following journalism's dictum "if it bleeds, it leads," most reporters focused on the study's shocking outcomes and failed to probe deeply into the data. But in fairness to the reporters, the language in the study itself, which was published in the *Journal of the American Medical Association* on July 17, 2002, suggested an open-and-shut case against the use of hormone replacement therapy:

> **Main Outcomes Measures.** The primary outcome was coronary heart disease (CHD) (nonfatal myocardial infarction and CHD death), with invasive breast cancer as the primary adverse outcome. A global index summarizing the balance of risks and benefits include the 2 primary outcomes plus stroke, pulmonary embolism (PE), endometrial cancer, colorectal cancer, hip fracture, and death due to other causes.[5]

One problem with understanding the data from the experiment centers on the difference between relative risks and absolute risks. The authors of the WHI study determined there was a 29 percent increase in coronary heart disease in the group that received estrogen plus progestin versus the women in the placebo group. Four years after the study was published, however, a researcher from the Department of Molecular and Cellular Biology, Baylor College of Medicine, was among those scrutinizing the data and coming up with contrasting conclusions. In "A critique of Women's Health Initiative Studies (2002-2006)," James Clark explained how WHI had arrived at its numbers and then provided another interpretation of the data that focused on relative risk:

> Relative risk can be misleading and many people do not realize that the actual increases are very small and may be insignificant. The actual % increase [in coronary heart disease] is 0.07% . . . many authors agree that unless a hazard ratio is 3.0 or higher it is of no consequence. Therefore, by this standard, all of the hazard ratios in this study would be considered insignificant.[6]

Clark examined risk ratios for most of the adverse health effects cited in the WHI study, but he also notes that the published study does not contain enough information to run accurate numbers on some of them.

Another problem of interpretation relates to the participants—the 16,608 menopausal and postmenopausal women aged fifty to seventy-nine years recruited by forty US clinical centers. The question that went unexplored when results popped into the headlines was: How much does the composition of the study group affect the outcome of this research?

The women who participated were, for the most part, twelve to fifteen years past the onset of menopause; the average age of participants was sixty-three years. Because of that, none of them would have had premenopausal levels of estrogen and progesterone. In terms of health, that means their bodies had already undergone changes in organ and metabolic function that set the stage for certain diseases. A prime example is heart disease, as hormones produced by the ovaries play an important role in vascular health. As researchers were able to confirm shortly after the WHI study, if a woman in the study had already begun to experience the effects of vascular disease, pumping up her hormones to a premenopausal level would not have reversed it. The work of Wake Forest Medical School's T. B. Clarkson, discussed later in this chapter, was a definitive study on the subject. It was one of several concluding that maintaining hormonal levels instead of letting them drop can continue to protect many women from the onset of such disease.

HORMONE THERAPY THROUGH THE YEARS

Some form of HT has been around since the 1940s. Wyeth-Ayerst first introduced conjugated equine estrogens (estrogen from a mare's urine) as Premarin in 1941 in Canada and in 1942 in the United States. It was not until 1960, however, that popularity of estrogen therapy skyrocketed—and then plummeted in the mid-1970s, and then skyrocketed again until the WHI results made headlines in the early 2000s.

Not surprisingly, pharmaceutical companies funded the drive to convince women and their physicians that estrogen was the fountain of youth. This statement is not offered as a judgment, but rather as an insight into what was perceived as an opportunity to stay young—an opportunity that many women found valid and continue to find valid today.

Pamphlets in doctors' waiting rooms, feature articles in women's magazines, and a must-have book prompted estrogen prescriptions to double between 1960 and 1975. Although it was not known at the time, Wyeth-Ayerst funded the work of Dr. Robert A. Wilson, and that financial backing enabled him to produce a sensational paper in 1963 and a sensational bestselling book called *Forever Feminine* in 1966. It also paid the bills for the Wilson Research Foundation, which had its offices on Park Avenue in Manhattan.[7] At the time, Wilson had strong credentials, serving as part of the Department of Obstetrics and Gynecology of the Methodist Hospital of Brooklyn.

Wilson's paper, published in the *Journal of the American Geriatrics Society*, bore the disturbing title "The Fate of the Nontreated Post-Menopausal Woman: A Plea for the Maintenance of Adequate Estrogen from Puberty to the Grave." Written with his wife Thelma, a registered nurse, the article argues that estrogen deficiency causes preventable diseases—preventable only through estrogen therapy. Some of these medical issues are elevated levels of low-density lipoprotein cholesterol ("bad" cholesterol), hypertension, osteoporosis, impairment of carbohydrate metabolism, depression, "dry, scaly and inelastic" skin, myriad endocrine disorders, nervous system imbalances, and breast and genital changes.[8]

The Wilsons argued that a sixty- or seventy-year-old woman should not be denied the hormonal advantages of a woman who is twenty or thirty years old. They reasoned that replacing a hormone the ovaries are no longer able to make is like a diabetic replacing the insulin her pancreas fails to make. The Wilsons ask: "Why should she be denied therapy? Who is to decide the age of denial?"[9] They ultimately conclude that, "A beneficial estrogen level should be continued throughout life."[10]

A 1965 paper in the *Journal of the American Medical Association* captured the enthusiasm for estrogen therapy in the gynecologic community and even surfaced in medical school textbooks:

> In current medical and lay literature, a number of authors have expressed opinions on the necessity for continuous estrogen treatment in women. Some believe that for physiological and cosmetic reasons every woman should receive routine estrogen therapy throughout life and not only at menopause or when clinically indicated. Pleas have been made for adequate estrogen therapy from "puberty to grave." . . . The menopause would thus be eliminated and femininity would be preserved. On the heel of these publications a pharmaceutical company responded with an energetic sales promotion to acquaint physicians with their hormone products. Working regimens were outlined for cyclic replacement therapy.[11]

By 1975, Premarin had become the fifth-leading prescription drug in the United States.[12] Then came the first crash in popularity and sales. A link between estrogen therapy and endometrial cancer made the headlines.

Shortly after that, the big result of new clinical studies was that adding progesterone to therapy averted the problem. Hence, we started to see therapies formulated for women with a uterus containing progesterone, also known as progestin. Progesterone's big job is to regulate the condition of the lining, or endometrium, of the uterus.

Once again comfortable that threats presented by estrogen supplementation had been addressed, women resumed their enthusiasm for HT. Supported by massive advertising touting the value of estrogen in preventing osteoporosis, the message that HT was "safe again" got through to women. Sales in the 1980s soared.

Riding the wave of popularity, the makers of Premarin took their agenda up a notch in 1990. Wyeth approached the US Food and Drug Administration about labeling their product as protective against heart disease. The preventative benefits of estrogen related to heart disease were also championed by many in the medical community. The American College of Physicians ultimately suggested that women at high risk of heart disease consider taking estrogen after menopause.[13]

The National Women's Health Network loudly questioned the available data, which was based on observation rather than randomized controlled studies. In such studies, patients are divided into groups randomly; each group takes either the medication under scrutiny or a placebo. The Network's push-back got reinforcement from women's organizations that found the associated fountain-of-youth messaging offensive.

A groundswell of support for a serious, significant study of the effects of HT on women's health led female Members of Congress to make it a legislative issue. Congress ended up budgeting money for research and the result was the WHI study funded by the National Institutes of Health.

What happened next was covered in the opening section of this chapter. The poorly designed WHI study doomed HT for years to come; the effect of the bad news continues to this day.

TYPES OF HORMONE THERAPY

HT is not a single entity like aspirin. There are different combinations of hormones available and different delivery methods. The first distinction to be made is the difference between synthetic hormones and bioidenticals.

Synthetic hormones are chemical substances produced in laboratories that are supposed to mimic the function of hormones produced by the body. They differ in structure from the naturally occurring hormones, however. A common example is the estrogen in Premarin, which is sourced from pregnant female horse's urine. It is a good match for a human woman's estrogen, but not exactly the same. The first synthetic estrogen was apparently described in a report published in 1933.[14]

Many young women are probably familiar with synthetic progesterone, called progestin. They may not know the name medroxyprogesterone acetate; however, they may have heard of brand names such as Depo-Provera, which is a popular and effective contraceptive. As part of hormone therapy in menopause, progestin protects a woman's uterus from the thickening that might predispose her to uterine cancer.

Synthetic testosterone is a substance many men know because it is used to treat hypogonadism (low testosterone). Bodybuilders—men and women—also have relied on it for decades to get the super-muscled look, like Arnold Schwarzenegger. (Interestingly, he relied on other performance-enhancing drugs; synthetic testosterone was hard to get when he was at his peak in the early to mid-1970s.) Androgen therapy, or the administration of testosterone for medical reasons, is used for menopausal women to treat symptoms such as low sexual desire, low sexual satisfaction, fatigue, and even depression.

Bioidentical hormones, as defined by Harvard Medical School, are

> hormones that are identical in molecular structure to the hormones women make in their bodies. They're not found in this form in nature but are made, or synthesized, from a plant chemical extracted from yams and soy. Bioidentical estrogens are 17 beta-estradiol, estrone, and estriol. (Estradiol is the form of estrogen that decreases at menopause.) Bioidentical progesterone is simply progesterone. It's micronized (finely ground) in the laboratory for better absorption in the body.[15]

HTs do not necessarily use one or the other. Sometimes they are combined in a product. Insights and stories on the relative risks and benefits are woven throughout the discussion that follows.

The Harvard analysis of synthetics and bioidenticals gives an even-handed, and amply supported, evaluation of how the body processes both:

> Technically, the body can't distinguish bioidentical hormones from the ones your ovaries produce. On a blood test, your total estradiol reflects the bioidentical estradiol you've taken as well as the estradiol your body makes. On the other hand, Premarin is metabolized into various forms of estrogen that aren't measured by standard laboratory tests. Proponents of bioidentical hormones say that one advantage of bioidentical estrogen over Premarin is that estrogen levels can be monitored more precisely and treatment individualized accordingly. Skeptics counter that it hardly matters, because no one knows exactly what hormone levels to aim for, and symptoms, not levels, should be treated and monitored.[16]

The following section on the controversy over bioidenticals details why some physicians are vocal opponents of them despite the fact that they are identical to hormones naturally produced in the body.

In addition to the differentiation between synthetic and bioidentical, the type of HT can also be looked at in terms of what single hormone, or combination of hormones, plays a role in the therapy:

1. Estrogen-only therapy, which is prescribed for women who have had a hysterectomy.
2. Estrogen-plus-progesterone therapy, which is given to women with a uterus to protect them against uterine (endometrial) cancer. Giving estrogen alone to these women creates cancer risks.
3. One of the above plus androgen therapy.

HT can be given with systemic products that are ingested or administered through a patch, injection, gel, emulsion, cream, or spray. They are designed to mitigate the whole-body symptoms noted in the last chapter, such as hot flashes and bone density. Nonsystemic products would include vaginal creams, rings, or tablets; their use is targeted specifically at relieving vaginal and vulvar symptoms. Examples include the following:

- Estrogen cream, such as Premarin, is applied in cycles, with the usual cycle being twenty-one days of continuous use followed by a week off. The same cautions that apply to the administration of systemic estrogen-only therapy apply here.

- A vaginal pessary is a device, often a ring, that is inserted into the vagina. It releases estrogen over time.
- Estradiol tablets come packaged in an applicator, which is inserted into the vagina; pressing the plunger releases the tablet.
- Pellets containing estradiol or testosterone that are implanted.

Pellet implantation comes with a special caution. Pellets a little bigger than the size of a grain of rice are implanted into subcutaneous tissue— tissue that has fewer blood vessels than other parts of the body—such as in the hip, underarm, or stomach area. They are supposed to provide an even release of hormones, dissolving over a period of a few months. Unfortunately, the pellets are not likely to release hormones evenly, and if there is a problem with too high a dose, you are stuck with it.

One physician who contributed to this book told me the story of a woman who made an emergency appointment with her to remove a testosterone pellet that had been implanted just weeks before by another doctor. The dose was so high, the woman had developed a serious problem with facial hair. Unfortunately, the physician had to break the bad news: The woman would simply have to wait until the pellet completely dissolved over the next couple of months. There was no way to remove it.

Pills and creams may require daily action on the part of a patient, but that action can be aborted at the first indication of overdose. Pellets are popular because they do not require daily maintenance, but the risk of a bad result may not be worth the convenience.

THE CASE FOR HORMONE THERAPY

Rebecca Dunsmoor-Su, a practicing gynecologist in the Seattle area who specializes in menopause, offers this on the pro side of HT:

> Hormone therapy is a good thing on balance. A lot of women are scared of it and very worried about risk. But the relative risk of most bad outcomes is very low. It can be the right treatment for a woman, but slowly but surely, other non-hormonal things are coming out in the market, mostly for vaginal symptoms. I wish we had more options for the systemic symptoms like hot flashes and night sweats. A lot of the other things we have to offer just don't work as well as hormones. For those symptoms, hormones work the best.[17]

Hundreds of clinical studies document the benefits of systemic HT in addressing conditions such as hot flashes, vaginal dryness, night sweats, and bone loss.[18] A menopausal woman who started HT at an early stage of her transition and is a good candidate for the therapy because of her health history can enjoy improved sleep and sexual relations, as well as an overall upgrade in her quality of life.

Joan had been a sound sleeper her whole life until she hit her mid-forties. At first, she attributed the problem to the chaos in her life—having three teenagers at home, a full-time job, and a husband who worked as a physician by day and a musician by night. Eventually, it occurred to her that her new restlessness at night might be due to the onset of menopause, so she contacted her OB-GYN. The doctor suggested HT.

> There was a lot of hoopla about how good hormone therapy was for the heart and bones, and my doctor thought it might eliminate the problem I was having getting to sleep and staying asleep. I was working as a government lawyer at the time and we had an abundance of support at the office about doing it, too.[19]

Joan's OB-GYN had delivered two of her three children, so she had known the doctor for many years and trusted her completely. The doctor put her on Activella, relatively low-dose tablets that had just been approved in 2000 when Joan was turning forty-seven years. Activella (generic name: estradiol, norethindrone acetate) contains both estrogen and progestin. Taken once a day, each tablet contains 1 mg of estrogen (17 beta-estradiol and is bioidentical) and 0.5 mg of progestin (norethindrone acetate, which is a synthetic hormone).

> It was amazing! I could sleep through the night, had no hot flashes, my vagina felt as young and lubricated as it ever had, my skin looked great. I had no problems at all—not from menopause or the hormones. My husband, who is a rheumatologist, was also very happy that I was doing something in addition to exercise to keep my bones healthy.

Her sister, who is two years older, had a different story. Plagued with hot flashes, she also tried HT but had to stop due to waves of vertigo. It was not a problem she had been warned about because HT is supposed to help alleviate problems like dizziness rather than bring it on.

The sister gave up on HT in a matter of months, but Joan stayed on her "baby dose," as she calls it, for almost fifteen years. When her doctor saw how well Joan responded to it during the first couple of years, she said she could stay on it for the rest of her life if she wanted—and Joan was tempted. Most of the women she knew socially, who were generally early fifties to mid-seventies, were on HT. She noticed they looked younger and stronger than other women their age, and she was among them.

Her reason for going off HT had nothing to do with problems or fears, and everything to do with inconvenience. She had developed a benign cyst, so every time she had a mammogram, which was every year, Joan was told to get a second screening "to be sure." She found herself driving to a specialist who was well-regarded, but geographically undesirable.

Without consulting her doctor, Joan blamed the HT for the mammography issues and decided to wean herself from the tablets. She dropped from once a day to two a week to once a week and then stopped.

I'm not sure I should have gone off of it. When you're out of estrogen, unpleasant things happen. Skin, bones, sleep—it seems they just go to hell and the hormones prevented that. I play a lot of tennis, but my weight is now an issue. And I've dried up inside. It's much more of a fight to stay young looking and young feeling than it was when I was on the hormones. Maybe I shouldn't have gone off them.

Joan was on HT throughout the years when the frightening headlines warned that taking estrogen could cause cancer, clots, stroke, and other horrible outcomes. She was fully aware that people who knew she was on HT were worried about her. But all those years, she had checkups and screenings, exercised regularly, and felt fabulous. Her experience is part of a large body of both anecdotal and scientific evidence that a woman who is a good candidate for HT can reap substantial benefits.

Thomas B. Clarkson of the Wake Forest University School of Medicine set out to study one of the primary alleged benefits of early estrogen therapy in his work with primates. His focus: premenopausal estrogen deficiency with resulting premature coronary artery atherosclerosis. Robert Wool, founder of the Women's Health Associates in Massachusetts where he has been in practice as an OB-GYN for thirty years, cites Clarkson's research as a primary piece of scientific evidence that HT can have undeniable health benefits when administered properly. In layman's terms, Wool explains what Clarkson did with his monkeys:

> He took the ovaries out of the monkeys to make sure there was no estrogen. He gave those monkeys a terrible diet, known to cause heart disease and atherosclerosis, and they got heart disease. What a surprise! Then he took the ovaries out of other monkeys, but gave them estrogen at the same time he gave them a horrible diet and none of them got heart disease.
>
> Then he took another group of monkeys with no ovaries, gave them a rotten diet for four years and *then* gave them estrogen. Well, the longer you wait, the more heart disease there is.[20]

Clarkson's published findings summarized the results as follows:

> Monkey studies have provided convincing evidence for the primary prevention of coronary artery atherosclerosis when estrogens are administered soon after the development of estrogen deficiency. Equally convincing are the data from monkey studies indicating the total loss of these estrogens beneficial effects if treatment is delayed for a period equal to six postmenopausal years for women.[21]

The message on HT from research like Clarkson's is this: If you want to commit to HT, do it early.

CONTROVERSY OVER BIOIDENTICAL HORMONES

Bioidenticals are hormones that are chemically identical to the hormones your body is producing or once produced. As noted previously, bioidenticals for estrogen—specifically estradiol, the form of estrogen that declines at menopause—are 17 beta-estradio, estrone, and estriol. The bioidentical for progesterone goes by the same name, and the same is true for testosterone.

The so-called natural bioidenticals come from plant or animal sources rather than being synthesized in a laboratory. (The concept of "natural" is tricky, however, as Premarin is not considered a bioidentical; it is synthetic estrogen, yet it comes from pregnant mares' urine.) Despite their natural origins, bioidenticals still make their way into a lab because they need to be processed for inclusion in a product. For example, soy and yam are the plant sources of estrogen in a drug called Estrace, which is manufactured by Allergan. But while Estrace is approved by the US Food and Drug Administration, a number of other supplements are not regulated, so it is anyone's guess exactly how much estrogen the woman taking them is actually getting.

Some companies purportedly customize the formula to meet a woman's hormone needs by using blood or saliva tests. However, from hour to hour and day to day, hormone levels change. The Women's Health Research Institute at Northwestern University cautions:

> Women who use custom compounds will not always get the proper dose. Products from compounding pharmacies are not subjected to the same high quality assurance standards that commercially available hormone therapies have to meet. Furthermore, the [US Food and Drug Administration] does not approve any custom compounds.[22]

In other words, the supposed customizing is not based on exact science or physiology. In addition, it seems currently that, regardless of how good the compounding pharmacy is, on a day-to-day basis, you will likely get different doses of hormones because of the difficulty of making each dose a perfect match for another one. Independent laboratory tests have shown a deviation of anywhere from 10 percent to 425 percent of the amount of hormone that the label indicates they are taking.[23] One big risk is that women taking these customized compounds do not know if they are getting enough progesterone to balance the estrogen, so the risk goes up for uterine cancer.

Without meaning to do any harm, Oprah Winfrey caused a surge in interest in bioidenticals when she talked about the positive physical and psychological effects of them—effects that she described as immediate.[24] Even though Winfrey did not recommend them to every woman, she "led by example," with the assumption being that someone as intelligent as she is, and with as many resources as she has, would not rely on an unsafe product.

In her online article "Bioidentical Hormones: Are They Safer?" Mayo Clinic physician Shannon K. Laughlin-Tommaso opens with a one word answer: "No." She continues:

> According to the Food and Drug Administration (FDA) and several medical specialty groups, the hormones marketed as "bioidentical" and "natural" aren't safer than hormones used in traditional hormone therapy, and there's no evidence they're any more effective.[25]

A study entitled "The Bioidentical Hormone Debate" concluded precisely the same thing: "According to the US Food and Drug Administration and The Endocrine Society, there is little or no evidence to support claims that bioidentical hormones are safer or more effective."[26]

Despite the apparent lack of enthusiasm and endorsement of bioidenticals in the medical community, science marches on and what may have been legitimate cautions when this book was written may not be sustainable by the time you read this. We are not trying to de-legitimize compounding pharmacies, but rather encourage more consistency in preparing formulas, as well as more clinical studies related to bioidenticals.

Different aspects of wellness expert Lori Ann King's struggles after her total hysterectomy, including her issues with bioidenticals, are woven throughout the book. Those of us who went through natural menopause had the advantage of being forewarned—for years—about the effects and possible ways to deal with them. Many women like Lori, however, woke up from surgery and unexpectedly had a doctor talking to her about systemic HT versus localized HT versus bioidenticals in various forms versus nothing at all. In pain, on pain medicine, confused, and sad, a woman is forced to start making choices that will likely affect her day-to-day life for months or even years to come.

After sorting out the options, Lori chose bioidentical HT (BHRT), which her doctor prescribed at her first checkup a week after her surgery. She immediately began applying daily creams of both estradiol, sourced from soy and yams, and progesterone to her skin. At first, the results disappointed her.

In her book *Come Back Strong*, which gives details of the mainstream and alternative therapies she tried, she talks about persistent, intense symptoms during the early days of BHRT. Returning to work particularly triggered her already serious mood swings. Colleagues of both genders did not empathize with her situation: this wasn't "just" an anticipated hysterectomy done robotically with hardly a scar. This was a procedure that abruptly removed most of her reproductive organs.

Six weeks after the surgery, she had a checkup with a doctor she had known prior to her surgery, and he happened to be an expert in BHRT. Over the course of the next year, he adjusted Lori's HT, increasing the doses based on reported symptoms and bloodwork. Throughout this time, she says all of the following went from "reported symptoms" to complaints:

hot flashes, night sweats, fatigue, insomnia, loss of libido, weight gain, lack of focus, zombie-like state, depression, anger, and overall lack of passion and energy for anything in life.

I learned that hormone therapy is not an exact science. In fact, it seemed a bit like a guessing game as we attempted to balance my hormones and emotions and help me feel good again. The hardest part, perhaps, was that it simply took time to get it right.[27]

Ultimately, through adjustments in dosages and even going off BHRT for a while, Lori concluded: "BHRT ended up having a positive effect on my quality of life. Although at first, it didn't feel like it."[28]

The situations of Joan and Lori illuminate the need for the individual woman to pay attention to what works for her and to communicate her thoughts and experiences to her doctor.

CAUTIONS ON HORMONE THERAPY

The primary cautions related to HT concern when a woman begins the therapy and how well-acquainted her physician is with her health and needs. A healthy woman beginning HT when she is in perimenopause has the basis for the best success. An older woman may not be as fortunate as the WHI study illuminated because of changes in health status that have already begun. A postmenopausal woman who has tested positive for the BRCA gene, predisposing her toward breast and ovarian cancer, may actually have a reduced risk of breast cancer with HT.[29]

There is one persistent caution and that is the link between estrogen-only therapy for a woman with a uterus and uterine (endometrial) cancer. The prescribing physician or physician's assistant needs to learn the distinction between estrogen-only and estrogen plus progesterone therapy. Some of us have had the unfortunate experience of being prescribed synthetic estrogen-only products and subsequently being diagnosed with uterine cancer.

The product itself can have tremendous benefits if it is a match for the needs and health status of the woman, but a woman may be the victim of the "fine print" in the warning literature if there is a mismatch.

Chapter Four

Intimacy and Wellness

Having just looked at options for fortifying levels of hormones that are depleted during menopause, it is time to consider how to boost production of other feel-good hormones. In some cases, there are both natural and pharmaceutical options.

SOURCE AND FUNCTION OF HORMONES

Hormones are chains of amino acids, and they are produced in the nine key endocrine glands: hypothalamus, pituitary gland, thyroid, parathyroids, adrenal glands, pineal body, pancreas, and the two reproductive glands (ovaries in a woman and testes in a man). In brief, the job of each is as follows[1]:

- Hypothalamus: Links the nervous and endocrine systems and controls the pituitary gland. You will see more references to this gland in relation to two of the feel-good hormones in this chapter, and then again in later chapters delving into the role of memory in sexual motivation.
- Pituitary glands: Control other endocrine glands and regulate processes including growth, blood pressure, and water balance. It also has a role in the release of some feel-good hormones in the body.
- Thyroid gland: Produces hormones such as thyroxine that controls energy-related reactions and other functions in cells.

- Parathyroid gland: Regulates the blood's calcium levels.
- Adrenaline glands: Release adrenaline, which triggers a response to emergencies or excitement. Other hormones from these glands affect salt and water balance in the kidneys and sugar in the blood. The adrenal glands are also a source of testosterone—the "libido hormone"—for both men and women.
- Thymus gland: Helps the immune system develop during childhood.
- Pancreas: Produces the hormones insulin and glucagon, which control the blood's glucose level.
- Testes: Release the hormone testosterone, which controls changes in a growing male's body and regulates sperm production. There is a great deal more discussion of testosterone in later chapters.
- Ovaries: Sources of your female reproductive hormones; by now, you are quite familiar with how they function. It should be noted that they produce testosterone, too, the supply of which diminishes with menopause.

Menopause puts particular stresses on the system, many of which we have looked at in depth. Those stresses can have negative ancillary effects besides primary symptoms such as hot flashes and night sweats. There is potentially a cascading biochemical effect that takes us deeper into an emotional and psychological black hole, where even the thought of intimacy is bothersome.

That's when we need intimacy the most—and sleep, and exercise, and a sense of accomplishment, and chocolate. We need to be active in our pursuit of activities and circumstances that stimulate production of happy hormones. We need to generate

- oxytocin,
- endorphins,
- serotonin, and
- dopamine.

These four hormones have multiple health benefits when we have appropriate amounts of them circulating in our system. The results are things like a strengthened immune system, reduced hot flashes, an ability to win the battle of anxiety and even depression, better sleep, weight loss, and a desire for sex as well as greater satisfaction having sex.

OXYTOCIN, INTIMACY, AND
THE IMMUNE SYSTEM

Oxytocin is the hormone most associated with loving touch and proximity to people we trust and with whom we share joy. Oxytocin begets oxytocin in that it enhances the desire for more interpersonal closeness and amplifies feelings of empathy. It is produced in the hypothalamus and secreted into the bloodstream by the pituitary gland—but only when cells in the hypothalamus are excited.

You currently cannot buy oxytocin the way you can buy hormone therapy, although a nasal spray has been created for studies focused on the hormone. Evidence suggests that MDMA (±3,4-methylenedioxy-methamphetamine) triggers the same effects as the hormone because the drug releases it. Commonly known as "Ecstasy"—although not all Ecstasy even contains MDMA anymore—this drug can't be bought legally, unless you are in Amsterdam. That may change in the United States, however, because federal government regulators have approved MDMA for use in large-scale clinical trials centered on treatment for post-traumatic stress disorder.[2] Why? It engenders a desire to interact with other people, to feel empathy, and to trust.

In the meantime, if we want more oxytocin, we have to make it ourselves. And it doesn't just make us happy: the presence of oxytocin means that we are nourishing our immune system. In other words, intimacy helps keep us healthy.

From the moment human beings are born to the moment we die, we need close relationships for both our physical and mental health. We get sick without the emotional security that flows from positive connections to other beings.

Intimacy—and I am not referring to penetrative sex here—can involve a lot of different tastes, flavors, and shapes, but it is necessary. Some women treat menopause as an excuse to back off from intimate relationships, as though their work as women is done and now they can retire to the privacy of their television room and not have to bother with being touched or touching. That's preparation for death, not life. That's preparation for sickness, not health.

From the disciplines of neurobiology, psychology, immunology, psychiatry, sociology, and radiology, we have learned that the health of our relationships—with physical contact—not only contributes to our quality of life, but also has the power to extend life itself.

Infants who are deprived of physical contact do not thrive. Their physical, psychological, and emotional issues were famously documented by psychologist John Bowlby, known as the "father of attachment theory." Bowlby's early 1950s research for the World Health Organization examined the health issues of homeless children who were deprived of maternal touch. There are also clinical studies involving adults that seem to prove we must have physical contact with other human beings in order to be healthy in all ways. Psychotherapist Sharon K. Farber made a compelling, research-based point in her 2013 article "Why We All Need to Touch and Be Touched" for *Psychology Today*. She stated:

> Being touched and touching someone else are fundamental modes of human interaction, and increasingly, many people are seeking out their own "professional touchers" and body arts teachers—chiropractors, physical therapists, Gestalt therapists, Rolfers, the Alexander-technique and Feldenkrais people, massage therapists, martial arts and T'ai Chi Ch'uan instructors. And some even wait in physicians' offices for a physical examination for ailments that have no organic cause—they wait to be touched.[3]

An experiment known as the "Still Face,"[4] conducted by Edward Tronick, director of the Child Development Unit at Harvard University, shows the heartbreaking result of a mother severing the connection with her infant for just two minutes. The experiment was first conducted in 1975 and was then repeated in 2009. The first scene shows a mother playing happily with her one-year-old baby. The infant smiles, points, and clearly interacts with her mother. The mother then turns away; when she faces the baby again, it is with a blank expression. Almost instantly, the baby responds to the difference. She uses all her ability to try to get the mother's attention again, first smiling and pointing, and then trying to reach her with both hands. She resorts to screeching, turning away, and sobbing uncontrollably. All the negative responses stop when the mother re-engages with the baby.

In the first part of the experiment, there is a synchronized play of expressions and connections in a relational loop—mommy smiles and baby smiles; baby points and mommy looks where baby is pointing. When we are in that patterned, rhythmic connection with one another, we are laying down positive neurological pathways in our brains. When that's cut off, it is painful. Watch the YouTube video[5] to see how much anguish just two minutes of disconnection causes the baby. The rhythmic response cycle in an adult relationship helps reinforce certain expectations related to that connection. So when we experience disconnection with our partner, we are like that baby. We may shut our feelings down for a moment, smiling and pointing, and try to cope with the loss. Alternatively, we might scream for attention. Both are signs of stress that may abate, but it will not go away until someone helps us re-establish a sense of emotional equilibrium through a positive connection. The connection primes the body for oxytocin production.

We can track the link between close relationships and immune system health back to the nineteenth century, so the association between intimacy and wellness is built on generations of research. In 1858, British epidemiologist William Farr pioneered this investigation when he began studying the "conjugal condition" of people in France. He didn't have the variety of types of couples we have today, of course; back then, you were married to someone of the opposite sex, single, or widowed. He was able to ascertain that people without ongoing relationships were at much greater risk for disease and death.

In an April 2010 article in the *New York Times*, health writer Tara Parker-Pope brought readers current on the work begun by Farr by spotlighting the latest research on the impact of intimate relationships on the immune system.

Contemporary studies, for instance, have shown that married people are less likely to get pneumonia, have surgery, develop cancer or have heart attacks. A group of Swedish researchers has found that being married or cohabiting at midlife is associated with a lower risk for dementia.[6]

The flip side of this is that a relationship plagued with problems has the opposite effect: It introduces health risks. It's only genuine intimacy engendering oxytocin production that carries with it substantial benefits for the immune system.

Psychiatrist Janice Kiecolt-Glaser, in conjunction with her colleagues in behavioral medicine and psychology at Ohio State University, closely studied the correlation between relationship status, health, and immune function. She makes powerful and very specific statements about the link, although we should expand her definition of "marital" to include any long-term intimate relationship:

> Marital relationships are strongly related to many aspects of physical health. Not only are married individuals healthier than single, divorced or separated and widowed individuals after controlling for income and age; marital status has substantial predictive power for mortality from a range of chronic and acute conditions. Compared to other social relationships, marital relationships tend to have a greater impact on an individual's emotional and physical well-being.[7]

The bottom line on boosting oxytocin production is this: When we are relaxed and feeling safe our bodies are able make more of it, and then the excitement of close contact triggers the release into the bloodstream. In that state, we are predisposed to be healthier. When we are stressed, under some kind of physical or psychological threat, we make hormones that wear down our immune system.

Cortisol is the main hormone that wreaks havoc with the adaptive immune system, a subset of the immune system designed to eliminate infectious agents or to at least prevent their growth. Basically, the cortisol surge as part of a fight-or-flight response breaks down tissues and increases the level of blood sugar. Along with adrenaline, it is a primary fight-or-flight hormone that races through the bloodstream as an automatic defense reaction. Cortisol helps prepare us to run away or throw something; it is not a feel-good hormone, but it is necessary for survival.

The stress you face that elevates the cortisol level and makes oxytocin a distant memory does not have to be a gun pointed at your head. It might be your teenager slamming the door after you criticize her new tattoo.

Menopause is a stressful time, with different degrees of stress experienced by each woman. The threats include loss of control, loss of youth, and uncomfortable symptoms. Making a conscious effort to reduce that stress and increase pleasure is a healthful, proactive step. One approach is hormone therapy, but there are others to boost your sense of control, aspects of youthfulness, and mitigation of symptoms. More on how to do that—and rev up your oxytocin production—in later chapters.

THE HEALTHY HIGH OF ENDORPHINS

Endorphins are a naturally produced opioid, meaning they help us handle pain, but we can get high on them, too. They can give us that lightheaded, walking-on-air feeling. The physical stress of exercise will get the endorphins going in our system. Doing that on a regular basis, even as little as a daily, thirty-minute walk, has been shown to have huge benefits for people suffering from depression. Both aerobic and anaerobic exercise activate endorphin production, one center of which is the pituitary gland.

Any menopausal woman who experiences mood swings and depressive episodes should get to the gym, go for a walk, or clean the house every day to get the endorphins going—whatever you feel motivated to do, do it regularly. And if none of those things appeal to you, you can go for the endorphin release by relying on acupuncture or massage therapy. Practicing meditation can also do it. Finally, having sex powers up your endorphin release. The benefits of having sex are that you get both the opioid and the oxytocin, of course.

The bitter reality is that if you are depressed, you are not inclined to exercise or have sex. Duly noted. Quite literally, take it a step at a time. Wearing a fitness tracker has helped so many women I know. Maybe your first day, a baseline day, is two thousand steps and you want to do ten thousand. Fine, take it to twenty-five hundred the next day and just keep moving up from there. And if you can convince a friend or two to wear the tracker and compare notes, that can help if you have a tiny competitive streak in you that serves as a motivator.

A study that looked at structured exercise and its benefits for depressed people had great news about endorphins. Of particular note is that research has suggested that the benefits of exercise in terms of mental health are long-lasting.

> The efficacy of exercise in decreasing symptoms of depression has been well established. Data regarding the positive mood effects of exercise involvement, independent of fitness gains, suggest that the focus should be on frequency of exercise rather than duration or intensity until the behavior has been well established.[8]

Don't become discouraged if you take a brisk walk or lift weights with a friend who feels better than you do afterward. Endorphin release is not identical for every person.

SEROTONIN SUNSHINE

Women going through menopause who also suffer from seasonal affective disorder experience a double whammy. One of the women interviewed for this book had that exact health challenge. Over the course of about eight years—the main portion of her menopause—she became severely depressed in the fall and winter.

Serotonin is the sunshine hormone, meaning that it makes you feel good and production of it is triggered by sunshine, among other things. Although it's commonly referred to as a hormone, it is considered a neurotransmitter, which is a chemical transmitting nerve impulses from one spot to another. Endorphins and dopamine are also considered neurotransmitters in addition to being labeled hormones.

Despite its designation as a brain neurotransmitter, an estimated 90 percent of your body's serotonin is made in the digestive tract and is known as "peripheral serotonin." Scientists have seen a link between low peripheral serotonin levels and irritable bowel syndrome, cardiovascular disease, and osteoporosis.[9] Menopausal women already face higher risk factors for the latter two, so paying attention to serotonin levels is particularly important later in life. Research indicates that certain bacteria in the gut contribute to the production of peripheral serotonin[10] and that getting sufficient dietary fiber stimulates the presence of that bacteria.[11]

Serotonin has not only been deemed important in treating depression, but also in diminishing susceptibility to depression and suicide.[12] It also helps nerve cells communicate and supports regulation of the body's sleep-awake cycles. Other functions, which are not as well documented, are probably a role in regulating appetite, as well as motor, cognitive, and autonomic functions. Perhaps its most impactful function, however, is on emotions, with the link between low serotonin levels and depression.

Serotonin cannot cross the blood-brain barrier (BBB). Serotonin used inside the brain must be produced inside the brain.[13] But serotonin can become a "victim" of other substances and circumstances affecting the integrity of the BBB.

Multiple teams of researchers have concluded that emotional, psychological, and environmental stress influence brain function. Specifically, stress causes a breakdown in the BBB, which separates blood circulating in your body from the brain fluid in your central nervous system. It prevents certain types of large molecules, such as bacteria, from flowing into the brain fluid, but allows others, such as hormones, to get through. The laboratory studies about the relationship between stress and brain dysfunction have been going on for decades but it wasn't until a key paper on the subject came out in 2010 that researchers concluded, "it appears that the BBB is the *gateway* to neuropsychiatric diseases."[14] Then they went on to discuss the effects of stress-induced brain dysfunction.

Your first order of business, therefore, is to try to reduce the stress in your life. Understandably, there is a chicken-egg situation in reducing stress and boosting the production of hormones that help you reduce stress. Menopause has its conundrums. Just keep the dark chocolate handy: Cacao boosts levels of serotonin.

Selective serotonin reuptake inhibitors (SSRIs) are antidepressants that are sometimes prescribed for menopausal women—not necessarily for depression or to reduce anxiety, though. SSRIs, as well as serotonin-norepinephrine uptake inhibitors, have been shown in clinical studies to reduce the severity and frequency of hot flashes.[15] (Norepinephrine is a neurotransmitter released by the adrenal gland and nerves of the sympathetic nervous system that constricts blood vessels, among other things.)

SSRIs inhibit the reabsorption, or reuptake, of serotonin in the brain. That blocking action, in turn, makes more serotonin available to the brain.

Now for the downside of SSRIs. Women who take them commonly have a problem with sexual dysfunction. A menopausal woman who already has lack of lubrication, low libido, and difficulty or inability climaxing will find those conditions exacerbated. The hot flashes may be gone or diminished, and a general feeling of well-being may sweep over a woman on SSRIs, but intimacy issues will likely get worse. The latest science is not encouraging about interventional strategies, either, listing them as "tolerance, titration dosage, substitution to another antidepressant drug and psychotherapy."[16]

In an endeavor to increase serotonin in the brain without SSRIs, consider the documented impact of environmental and lifestyle factors. One conclusion of research is that alterations in thought through meditation or some other positive-thinking effort influences serotonin levels. (It apparently also can influence dopamine levels,[17] the subject of the next section.) A second is that exposure to sunlight, or properly configured artificial light, can increase serotonin production. The woman referenced at the beginning of this section happened to be financially fortunate. From the time she was diagnosed with seasonal affective disorder in her forties, her husband would make it possible for her to take at least two weeks each winter to vacation in a tropical location to escape the overcast skies of New England. A third strategy is exercise, which has been proven time and time again to have antidepressive effects due to stimulation of "happy hormones."

In addition to exposure to sunshine, therefore, positive thinking and exercise stimulate production of serotonin in the brain. Combine that with dietary fiber and foods like eggs, cheese, pineapples, salmon, nuts, and turkey, and you are on your way to having more serotonin circulating in your body.[18]

An important thing for your sex life is to keep serotonin in balance with the next hormone, dopamine.

THE REWARDS OF DOPAMINE

Dopamine is another neurotransmitter, or "messenger chemical," and it is associated with cravings and the subsequent reward of giving in to the desire. When you want to play blackjack and then sit down for a game, dopamine kicks in. When you win the game, you generate even more. When you are staging a once-in-a-lifetime dinner party—like your only daughter's wedding reception—you have a massive emotional investment and yearning to be praised. When the first guest says, "This is the most exquisite reception ever!" the dopamine is flooding your body. When you want sex and have it, same thing. Dopamine is made in a couple of different areas of the brain and released by the hypothalamus.

You also get a small boost of dopamine if you're a nice person. When you help a mom struggling to carry groceries and a baby at the same time, you get a tiny rush of dopamine. Acts of kindness in your daily life give you pleasure because you stimulate the production of dopamine. That is the biochemical reason why you would feel so good volunteering to dish out hot meals to people struggling with homelessness on Thanksgiving Day. Research suggests that even thinking about expressing love engenders dopamine production, so meditation and daydreaming can give you a little high. I have a friend who is a retired minister and occasionally preaches at the local Episcopal church—and she's brilliant! Every time she delivers another compelling, story-based message on Sunday, I can guarantee that the smiles and wide eyes in the congregation give her a big rush of dopamine.

Cacao also appears to have value in increasing your body's supply of dopamine. Although there is some difference of opinion as to the exact effect, there is evidence that cacao influences production of it.

Back in 1995, the authors of a paper called "Dopamine and Sexual Behavior" opened with the sentence: "Among central neurotransmitters involved in the control of sexual behavior, dopamine is certainly one of the most extensively studied."[19] Although that suggested something like, "We know a whole lot about this," the conclusion of the abstract indicated that researchers felt they had a handle on the role of dopamine in male sexual behavior, but that was not the case with how dopamine affected women.

> In contrast, no conclusion can be deduced from the available studies on the role of central dopaminergic systems in the control of proceptivity and receptivity, the two main components of female sexual behavior.[20]

Twenty years after that study was published, the US Food and Drug Administration approved flibanserin, a drug to improve female sex drive. It raises levels of dopamine and norepinephrine, and it reduces the amount of serotonin in the body. The intended outcome is to help a *premenopausal* woman with low sexual desire have the right balance of hormones to want to have sex. Clearly, focus on the issue posed in the 1995 paper yielded some increased understanding about the role of dopamine in female sexual behavior. Unfortunately, not enough under-standing. Studies indicated that flibanserin (marketed as Addyi) helped many women have more satisfying sex, but it did not do the one thing it was supposed to do: make them want more sex.[21]

Prior to US Food and Drug Administration approval, flibanserin was also investigated as a possible aid for *postmenopausal* women with low sexual desire. The researchers saw "significant improvements with flibanserin versus placebo"[22]; however, the drug was ultimately ap-proved only for premenopausal women.

Flibanserin received some good press, but in general the response from media and the marketplace was lukewarm. The manufacturer, Sprout Pharmaceuticals, also had myriad problems in getting the drug into the hands of women. It was very expensive (eight hundred dollars for a monthly prescription), was not stocked by most pharmacies, and physicians had little awareness of it. Sprout relaunched the product in June 2018 at a much lower price.

In the meantime, some researchers went back over their data and found there was evidence that the drug had an unexpected benefit for both premenopausal and postmenopausal women—something not directly related to sex drive. At least one study found strong evidence that it helped them lose weight.

The team led by Dr. Susan Kornstein of the Department of Psychiatry and the Institute for Women's Health at Virginia Commonwealth University had conducted one of the many studies focused on flibanserin's effect on hypoactive sexual desire disorder, which is what the drug was designed to treat. The study group included both premenopausal and postmenopausal women. When they looked at all the data they collected on the women, they found surprising, long-term weight loss:

> This retrospective analysis showed that treatment with flibanserin 100 mg qhs in women with [hypoactive sexual desire disorder] was associated with statistically significant weight loss compared with placebo in both premenopausal and postmenopausal patients. Weight loss without apparent weight regain was also observed during longer term, open-label flibanserin treatment of up to 18 months. In contrast to more typical serotonergic antidepressants, weight gain does not appear to be a clinical concern with flibanserin.[23]

The association of dopamine and weight loss is not new, although the flibanserin study called attention to a pharmaceutical way to address the problem of too many pounds. It had the added benefit of documenting long-term effects.

Dopamine—the hormone of desire and reward—actually helps you *beat* food cravings as long as you have a sufficient amount in your system. If your dopamine levels plummet, your body sends signals to the brain that compel you to satisfy your desire to eat. You grab something immediately.

> Low levels of dopamine dampen your dopamine receptors and lead you to lose control of your diet and what you eat. As your dopamine levels deplete, your food cravings will return because the body needs to have stabilized levels of the chemical in order to proactively prevent food binging. The feel-good mood you associate with sweets, sugars, and carbohydrates triggers "reward" networks in the brain that can be difficult to reverse.[24]

Considering what we know about producing the four feel-good hormones featured in this chapter, it seems we should all behave more like little kids—running and jumping in the sunshine, raiding the Easter basket, hugging our friends, and daydreaming. Andrew Weil, famous for combining Western mainstream medicine with alternative practices into "integrative medicine," has a simple list of six actions to take to generate the hormones of happiness[25]:

1. Walk outside.
2. Listen to music.
3. Eat some dark chocolate.
4. Pet your companion animal.
5. Straighten up; adopt good posture.
6. Take a sniff of aromas like vanilla and lemon.

To get the most out of these recommendations, Weil recommends combining them: "Play some uplifting music as you walk, being conscious of keeping your shoulders and head held high."[26] And then have the chocolate, pet the cat, and take a whiff of a vanilla bean when you get home.

Chapter Five

Sexuality

Libido, Motivation, and Culture

The concept of sexuality can be approached in at least three different ways: capacity for sexual feelings, sexual orientation or preference, and sexual activity. This chapter addresses only the first one, that is, the capacity for sexual feelings.

Betsy Cairo, a board-certified reproductive biologist and author of two textbooks, notes that the capacity for sexual feelings is not a purely physical ability. There are biological, psychological, and sociological aspects to reproductive health and human sexuality. It is important for people to understand themselves biologically and psychologically if they want to get a handle on their sexual functioning. Cairo adds: "The sociological part is what we're swimming in. It's our culture; it's everything around us. We want a balance of the triangle and the three elements can either work together to create that balance or work against each other."[1]

BIOLOGY AND LIBIDO

The biological component of sexual feelings is libido—the animal desire for sex. Libido tends to be much stronger when we're young. We have stamina as well as powerful hormones circulating in our body. We don't have to think about eating figs, bananas, avocados, and chocolate, which are all considered libido-boosting foods. And when we're young,

unless there is a medical problem, we don't have to worry about androgen hormone therapy.

Libido is a product of the "lower" brain systems responsible for animal urges and satisfaction. The psychology and culture components of
sexuality are tied to the "higher" brain system.

A physician at Yale Medical School named Paul D. MacLean took
us into the modern era of neuroscience in 1952 when he proposed the
"triune brain theory," meaning that the brain is actually three brains in
one. Today, we have a somewhat revised understanding of the brain's
structures, but the basic components identified by MacLean are still
used. They are known as the reptilian complex (reptilian brain), the
paleomammalian complex (the limbic system), and the neomammalian
complex (neocortex).

What's the importance of that? It represents how we evolved, with
libido not being a human function associated with thinking.

The reptilian complex controls involuntary survival functions, such as
heart rate and breathing. The fight-or-flight responses we have to a threat
emanate from this portion of the brain. Reproduction is part of survival,
so it should be noted that the libido starts here. From a physiological perspective, libido is controlled by the autonomic nervous system.

The limbic system, which emerged with mammals, is associated with
desires, emotions, and memory. The longing to have sex because of
emotional connection, euphoric memories, and anticipation of satisfaction might be called a "limbic libido." The limbic system would drive
us to want to repeat something we have found pleasurable and avoid an
activity that caused us pain.

The neocortex is the primate brain, and it is responsible for language,
imagination, learning, and consciousness. When philosopher and math-
ematician René Descartes asserted, "I think, therefore I am," he captured
the essence of what the neomammalian complex means to our humanity.

Unless you're a young adult and don't yet have a fully formed brain,
libido can be kept in check by the cognitive part of the brain—the
"higher self" that supposedly distinguishes us as human. Another
exception might be someone whose brain isn't functioning normally.
Science writer Carl Zimmer described three fascinating examples in the
opening of his article "The Brain: Where Does Sex Live in the Brain?
From Top to Bottom."[2] One case involved a fifty-four-year-old woman
diagnosed with nymphomania. In 1944, the treatment for that involved
blasting her ovaries with X-rays. That did nothing to mitigate her crav-

ings because the problem stemmed from a slow-growing brain tumor. Another case of apparent nymphomania arose in 1969, with the cause ultimately determined to be brain damage from syphilis. And even in this century, a woman in Taiwan baffled doctors with a complaint that brushing her teeth caused orgasm. The cause was epilepsy triggered by a swath of damaged brain tissue.

Zimmer explains that the case studies make a couple of things clear about the brain's involvement in sex:

> For starters, they demonstrate that sexual pleasure is not just a simple set of reflexes in the body. After all, epileptic bursts of electricity in the brain alone can trigger everything from desire to ecstasy. The clinical examples also point to the parts of the brain that may be involved in sexual experiences.[3]

Using functional magnetic resonance imaging (fMRI), scientists attempted to determined what parts of the brain that would be. Two components of the limbic system, the amygdala and hippocampus, figure prominently, and their functioning is explored in the next section. But the central conclusion of the research is that sexual arousal is associated with our highest brain function:

> The parts of the brain that light up in the fMRI scans include regions that are associated with some of our most sophisticated forms of thought. The anterior insula, for instance, is what we use to reflect on the state of our own bodies (to be aware of the sensation of butterflies in the stomach, say, or of lightness in the head). Brain regions that are associated with understanding the thoughts and intentions of other people also seem linked with sexual feelings.[4]

Knowing that your brain—from the part controlling your most primitive needs all the way up to the most sophisticated functions—plays myriad roles in your sex life; consider now the psychological component of your sexuality.

PSYCHOLOGY AND MOTIVATION

Betsy Cairo draws a sharp distinction between libido and sexual motivation. You might think of libido as needing or wanting, but sexual motivation as liking and enjoying.

> If you want to continue to have sex as you age, you need sexual motiva-
> tion. That is what will sustain you. Sexual motivation is a conscious effort
> to be physical, emotional, intimate with another person. Libido on the
> other hand is hormonally and instinct driven.
>
> Too many people think if they're not horny, or thinking about sex and
> wanting to have it—feeling the desire to scratch that itch—then there's
> something wrong with them. Maybe they have lost sight of the fact that
> the circumstances of their life make it impossible to be that charged up.
> Of course you would rather have ten minutes more sleep than sex if
> you're exhausted. But at that point, it's sexual motivation that puts you
> in the mood for sex. Suddenly, the ten minutes of extra sleep is inconse-
> quential to feeling a desire for loving touch.
>
> Libido can fail you, but sexual motivation will sustain you. It's a func-
> tion of making an effort.[5]

The unfortunate reality is that many people are too lazy to have sex.
They may blame physiology by saying they have no libido—and it is
true in some cases that the physical hunger just is not there—but it
could be a case of zero motivation.

If you can get yourself dressed to go to a dinner party, go shopping
for holiday gifts, show up at church, or go to the gym, you have made
conscious decisions to motivate yourself to take action. You can tap
into that ability to do a vast array of things to improve your intimate life.

When we treat our sex drive as something optional, something that
can be dispensed with, then we will let it wither. We can decide it is
too much trouble to read a book, so we just browse three hundred-word
articles that we can link to from the msn.com homepage. If we think
it's unnecessary to get exercise, why bother? It's no different with the
motivation to have sex: If we don't think sex is important, then the
desire will fade.

Consider what it might take to get up an hour earlier than you would
like to get some exercise. You may feel no motivation to do it, but your
yoga pants are at the foot of the bed on Monday morning when you
wake up. You see them. You put them on. You figure, "What the heck.
I'll go to the 7:30 yoga class today." The activity gets your endorphins
going and you feel great after the class and for the rest of the day. Tues-
day night, you put the pants out again because the classes are Monday,
Wednesday, and Friday. You wake up and see them and say, "What the
heck. I'll go to yoga today." Once again, you get the endorphins circulating, have a great day and put those feel-good yoga pants at the foot

of the bed on Thursday night. Friday morning, you wake up and find yourself looking forward to the 7:30 yoga class.

Sexual motivation can be similar. It's not just a matter of talking yourself into intimate moments with your partner, or saying you are doing it "for love." Instead, you plant a reminder—a reminder both to do it and to remind you of how good it feels to do it. Staying lubricated all the time through use of a vaginal moisturizer not only helps you stay healthy and prevent vaginal atrophy, but it is also an ongoing reminder that you have the ability to enjoy sexual intimacy at any time. It's a reminder of your ability to experience pleasure. You are manipulating the psychological aspect of your sexuality by reminding yourself that having arousing experiences, both through self-stimulation and with your partner, brings rewards.

The issue of rewards relative to motivation can be complicated, though. Sex educator and author (*Come As You Are*) Dr. Emily Nagoski covered this humorously in her April 2018 TED Talk, "The Truth about Unwanted Arousal."

You remember Pavlov? He makes dogs salivate in response to a bell. It's easy, you give a dog food, salivates automatically, and you ring a bell. Food, salivate, bell. Food, bell, salivate. Bell, salivate. Does that salivation mean that the dog wants to eat the bell? Does it mean that the dog finds the bell delicious? No. What Pavlov did was make the bell food-related. When we see this separateness of wanting, liking and learning, this is where we find an explanatory framework for understanding what researchers call arousal nonconcordance.

Nonconcordance, very simply, is when there is a lack of predictive relationship between your physiological response, like salivation, and your subjective experience of pleasure and desire. That happens in every emotional and motivational system that we have, including sex. Research over the last 30 years has found that genital blood flow can increase in response to sex-related stimuli even if those sex-related stimuli are not also associated with the subjective experience of wanting and liking. In fact, the predictive relationship between genital response and subjective experience is between 10 and 50 percent. Which is an enormous range. You just can't predict necessarily how a person feels about that sex-related stimulus just by looking at their genital blood flow. When I explained this to my husband, he gave me the best possible example. He was like, "So, that could explain this one time, when I was in high school, I . . . I got an erection in response to the phrase 'doughnut hole.'"[6]

In laywoman's terms, arousal nonconcordance means that you may be vaginally dry and highly aroused because of circumstances that stimulate your reward center. This could be especially true for a menopausal woman who wants sex, but her body doesn't support having penetrative sex. Alternatively, you might have no motivation for sex and yet, for some reason, be wet and appear to be ready. Again, with a menopausal woman, this could be stimulus-related, or you may just be well-prepared because of hormone therapy or vaginal moisturizers. It's a case of "looks can be deceiving." The mismatch is beyond your control, but the sexual motivation is the determining factor as to whether you are pleasure-bound.

Every sense can contribute to sexual motivation. (This is a theme that is explored with more of a how-to focus in chapter 7.) *Sense memory* can play a role in our drive to do anything. This is a phenomenon that lets us retain a distinct sense that we are still tasting, smelling, seeing, touching, or hearing something after the actual stimulus is no longer there. Smell has a particularly strong ability to provide sensory cues for emotions.

> Incoming smells are first processed by the olfactory bulb, which starts inside the nose and runs along the bottom of the brain. The olfactory bulb has direct connections to two brain areas that are strongly implicated in emotion and memory: the amygdala and hippocampus.[7]

The amygdala is a bit of gray matter that is part of the limbic system of the brain. It's a kind of processing center for the messages coming from our senses and internal organs. As mentioned before, the limbic system controls basic emotions like fear and pleasure, as well as memories and an innate sense of values. The hippocampus is also part of the limbic system. It puts the puzzle pieces of short-term memory together to give us long-term memories.

Without even realizing it, my partner Jim and I managed to use sense memory to transform my experience of chemotherapy. After almost six hours of sitting in a chair attached to a plastic pouch that was dripping life-saving toxins, one might assume I'd call the whole event "miserable." Quite the opposite. I wore my favorite pink shirt to the first session; it's a happy color, and the freshly washed shirt had a clean smell. Jim brought me some hot chicken soup and a bar of dark chocolate with raspberries. The aromas and tastes were incredibly soothing. We watched a funny show on television. As a bonus, my nurse had a beautiful smile and an outrageous sense of humor. Most importantly, Jim was there, bringing a loving presence into the room. I wouldn't call it a fun day, but I would assert that it was far from horrible.

It was his idea to wear the "lucky" pink shirt to the following sessions. He also repeated the soup and chocolate. Overall, the lingering memories I had of those sessions related to the sensory experiences rather than the medical treatment.

Sense memory can turn a potentially positive experience into something you think you want to avoid, too. An extreme example is a reluctance to touch or be touched after being sexually violated. A friend told me about a first, and last, date with someone she was very attracted to in college. They had the unfortunate experience of seeing an accident with a great deal of blood and smoke involved. On some level, they probably realized that another date would dredge up the vision of pain and suffering.

Just as Jim planted happy and soothing memories into my experience of chemotherapy, it is possible to "engineer" moments with your loved one that arouse happy sense memories. Hanging around together in the kitchen when aromas of roast beef and apple pie are in the air or having music you both enjoy in the background when you're puttering around the house—these are the little things that can warm up your desire to be together.

All types of memories, not just sense memory, can fuel sexual motivation. The challenge we all face is to form memories intentionally rather than just haphazardly. If we can learn to do that, then not only the quality of our memory mechanism will improve, but also the quality of the memories themselves will improve.

Joshua Foer is a science writer who immersed himself in the study of memory. He went to the US Memory Championship and discovered something astonishing: People who won memory contests were not necessarily super intelligent or even wired differently from most of us. A notable exception would be someone like Kim Peek, the savant on whom Dustin Hoffman's *Rain Man* character was based. Foer learned that people who won memory contests were generally not anything like that; they simply used and developed systems that they could teach other unexceptional people as well.

Foer started "working out" a little every day to train his memory. He went to the memory contest he had gone to the year before and thought, just for fun, that he would enter it. Much to his surprise, he won.

He shared a major insight of his year's sojourn into the study of memory in a TED Talk—and it's a message with great value for those who want more sexual motivation:

> We often talk about people with great memories as though it were some sort of an innate gift, but that is not the case. Great memories are learned. At the most basic level, we remember when we pay attention. We remember when we are deeply engaged. We remember when we are able to take a piece of information and experience, and figure out why it is meaningful to us, why it is significant, why it's colorful, when we're able to transform it in some way that makes sense in the light of all of the other things floating around in our minds.[8]

Memories are fuel for the imagination. We think back to a full-body spa treatment at a resort in Southern California and fantasize what it would have been like to have it become a happy-ending massage. We remember sharing an elevator with a sexy television star and imagine what might have happened if there were a sudden blackout that shut down the elevator for four hours.

Psychotherapist and relationship expert Esther Perel says, "A crisis of desire is a crisis of the imagination."[9] That statement reinforces what the researchers doing fMRI studies found: there is no sexual motivation without the involvement of the primate brain. The highly sophisticated part of our brain that enables us to communicate through language, design plans, and think abstractly has a vital role in sexual motivation. It is the center of imagination and, therefore, the center of our sexual desire.

SOCIOLOGY AND CULTURE

For purposes of this discussion, let's rely on this definition of culture: the attitudes and behavior characteristic of a particular social group. The dominant social group in our lives can have more influence than we realize, or wish to have, on the intimate part of our primary love relationship.

Let's play *Jeopardy!*

The answer is: a prince, an actress, a singer, a chief executive officer, a US president, a fire chief, and a tennis player.

The question is: Who were seven of *Time* magazine's 100 Most Influential People of 2018?

If *Time* did correctly identify the most influential people of 2018, then our cultural genetic material now contains bits of Prince Harry, Gal Gadot, Cardi B, Jeff Bezos, Donald Trump, West Virginia fire chief Jan Radar, and Roger Federer.

If we were overdramatizing the effect of such influencers on how we perceive ourselves and shape our relationships, we would all have a good laugh. The unfunny truth is that society, pop culture, and politics inform us about ways of relating to one another, about the expectations associated with relationships, and about what's acceptable behavior in a relationship versus what's something that elicits criticism. Add to that the influences of our family, the people in our professional and social circles, leaders in our religious organization, and others around us with whom we have regular contact.

As you read this section, ask yourself the question: Am I letting the influencers actually ruin my chances of finding connections and fulfillment because of how they affect my relationships?

In 2008, family sociologists Denise Donnelly and Elizabeth Burgess published a significant paper identifying factors that created the environment for a sexless marriage. The marriages they tried to understand involve what they called "involuntary celibacy" meaning that the couple did not make a mutual decision to refrain from sex, but rather circumstances drove them to it. One important conclusion was about social influences on sexuality:

> In terms of sexuality, social prescriptions also play a role. These include the social norms that committed couples remain sexually exclusive backed up by the legal norms that make it difficult for couples to end their relationship when it becomes less than satisfying.[10]

The researchers also noted that "the social supports of remaining together as a couple, if not a family, also keep the sexless couple together."[11]

Now, consider the flip side, which would be the minority in most modern cultures. This would be the couple who enjoys going on retreats offered by The Welcomed Consensus, a community that teaches how to succeed in relationships with fun as a goal. This is the couple that enjoys Esther Perel's video seminar on rekindling desire and feels comfortable talking about it with their friends. A couple like that has cultural reinforcement of a vibrant sexual life.

Cultural influences affect our intimate lives less overtly as well. Issues of self-image—am I attractive enough to deserve pleasure?—and romantic ideals can plague one or both members of a couple.

Too Much Focus on Externals

Society tells us whatever is on the outside is the truth—handsome, beautiful, talented, stylish, or just the opposite. Don't jump to conclusions about the sources of those messages, though. It isn't just media that reinforces our focus on the superficial. Without even meaning to, parents and pastors can "train" children to project virtue by hiding their vices; they look like "good" people, even when they hop over to the other side of the moral fence.

A humorous part of Hollywood lore is how many fine actresses weren't taken seriously until they "uglified" themselves for a role. "What you see is what you get" had condemned them, at least to some extent, to the perception that their primary value to movies was their attractiveness. Charlize Theron, Halle Berry, Nicole Kidman, and Hilary Swank (who did it twice) are among the beautiful actresses who forced us to look past their pretty surface, and they won Academy Awards for it.

In terms of relationships, keeping our attention on externals does to our friendships and other love relationships what Hollywood ostensibly did to those actresses: prevents them from giving us their best and blocks us from knowing what depth they have to offer.

After losing his wife, an acquaintance of mine joined a dating website and began trolling for blonde women who were considerably younger than him. In consideration of some of the non-physical traits he'd listed as desirable, he was matched with a classy, fit, grey-haired woman who was also in her mid-sixties. As he sat at dinner with her on their first date, he found himself forgetting that he'd been trolling for a younger woman. Three years later, they are still together. She had also experienced the loss of a spouse of more than thirty years, so they shared an understanding of commitment and enthusiasm for the chance to have a sex life again. When I hear stories like this, I get the urge to hug the people who design the software for some of these dating sites.

In his book, *Situations Matter: Understanding How Context Transforms Your World,* social psychology researcher Sam Sommers notes that we tend to take our context for granted and in doing so, we often accept that what we see is what we get. We like to minimize the amount of effort it takes to make decisions and make snap judgments about people because it just takes less brain power.

Just as bad, we make snap judgments about *ourselves* because of what we look like, how and where we were raised, and how we spend our days. We make snap judgments about our worthiness for affection and attention.

The Grant Study provides hard evidence that focusing on externals does not serve us well in terms of achievement or relationships. The positive physical effects of a secure relationship do powerful and practical things for our bodies and our sense of risk-taking and competence. The Grant Study began in 1938 and involved two populations of white males, one of which was a group of 268 Harvard University students. The research team did bi-annual follow-up through questionnaires, information from participants' physicians, and personal interviews, and kept track of participants still living until they were well into their nineties.

New York Times columnist David Brooks focused on one aspect of the Grant Study in an article entitled "The Heart Grows Smarter."

> In the 1930s and 1940s, the researchers didn't pay much attention to the men's relationships. Instead, following the intellectual fashions of the day, they paid a lot of attention to the men's physiognomy. Did they have a "masculine" body type? Did they show signs of vigorous genetic endowments?
>
> Body type was useless as a predictor of how the men would fare in life. So was birth order or political affiliation. Even social class had a limited effect. . . . As George Vaillant, the study director, sums it up in "Triumphs of Experience," his most recent summary of the research, "It was the capacity for intimate relationships that predicted flourishing in all aspects of these men's lives."[12]

Even with the preponderance of evidence reminding us to look past externals, we look for easy ways to understand each other and ourselves time after time. Externals do tell us something about people, but generally, they are like the proverbial tip of the iceberg: only 15 to 20 percent of the total.

The quality of our relationships is what affects our health and well-being, and that is not shaped by whether someone has made a fashion faux pas or pays for dinner with a platinum credit card.

One of the facts that surfaced through the years in the Grant Study is that, as Brooks suggests in the title of the piece, the hearts of the men assumed more significance in their health and happiness than their looks or degrees. They found that being the rogue or loner was a miserable way to live—that is, those who actually did live to realize it. Brooks makes it abundantly clear what happened to the others: "Of the 31 men in the study incapable of establishing intimate bonds, only four are still alive. Of those who were better at forming relationships, more than a third are living."[13]

Fairytale Distortions

The marriage of Meghan Markle and Prince Harry of Great Britain captivated the world. Millions of Americans rose early that day to watch an American commoner suddenly become a member of the royal family.

We could collectively sigh, "See? Fairytales do come true!" Some in the United States had let that sigh out a dozen years earlier when Katie Holmes married Hollywood royalty Tom Cruise, the man she'd had a crush on as a child. These relationships seem to validate our not-so-secret belief that make-believe stories do come true.

We drill the fairytale mentality into girls from an early age, as Peggy Orenstein, well-known for writing about issues affecting women and girls, notes in *Cinderella Ate My Daughter*. Orenstein was shocked when her daughter seemed transformed after a week of preschool:

"She came home having memorized, as if by osmosis, all the names and gown colors of the Disney princesses."[14] Her daughter also developed a thirst for pink, from dresses to a Magic 8-ball.

But the worst part was the messages about what to be: "And what was the first thing that culture told her about being a girl? Not that she was competent, strong, creative, or smart, but that every little girl wants—or should want—to be the Fairest of Them All."[15]

This fairytale view of ourselves and our relationships can persist not only through high school, but until (and even after) we're postmenopausal women. We can hit menopause and still see ourselves in some ways as a Disney princess who *ought* to be living happily ever after. When that gets in the way of seeing that our crow's feet and thirty-year marriage are signs of a mature fairytale, we let culture sabotage the possibilities for our intimate life.

The mix of psychological, emotional, and physical elements that compose sexuality is like a French cassoulet: It is a vat of ingredients, rich, meaty, and overwhelmingly simple—but give it time and it leads to supreme satisfaction!

Chapter Six

Finding a New Normal

Physical Needs

The physical and psychological changes of menopause can profoundly affect the quality of intimate relationships. This chapter addresses ways to mitigate or eliminate the systemic and vaginal physical symptoms in non-hormonal ways, with the psychological ones being the focus of chapter 7.

In *Sex and Cancer*, Dr. Saketh Guntupalli and I spotlighted the practical ways that women who have experienced sexual dysfunction after cancer treatment can enjoy a "new normal" both physically and psychologically. Everyone agrees that cancer tends to be a major life disrupter, but for many women, so is menopause! Much of the same advice we vetted and shared, therefore, also applies here.

The same issues of desire, comfort, and satisfaction that apply to a woman who has gone through cancer treatment apply to a woman who has gone through the normal transition, or through a surgical inducement, of menopause. The same stories about self-esteem, vaginal dryness, low libido, insomnia, hot flashes, and diminished pleasure come from women who have enjoyed good health throughout their lives but now find themselves in menopause or postmenopause.

The chapter features very specific guidance on finding a physical "new normal" as well as stories of couples who have enjoyed a resurgence of sexual activity during and after menopause. Although many parts of the body are discussed and explored in relation to how they play a role in rejuvenation of intimacy after menopause, there is a bit more emphasis on the vagina and vulva than other parts. The reason is that this is the area of the body hit hardest by the drop in estrogen production that comes with menopause.

Eve Ensler is a great inspiration in talking about this area of a woman's body. She is the author of *The Vagina Monologues* and engaged mid-life celebrities such as actors Whoopie Goldberg and Susan Sarandon to bring the original version of her play to life more than two decades ago. In the play, she offers what might be called vaginal inspiration for every reader of this book:

> The heart is capable of sacrifice. So is the vagina. The heart is able to forgive and repair. It can change its shape to let us in. It can expand to let us out. So can the vagina. It can ache for us and stretch for us, die for us and bleed and bleed us into this difficult, wondrous world. So can the vagina. I was there in the room. I remember.[1]

Many contributors to this book have described their attempts to mitigate symptoms of menopause to find or rediscover vibrant intimacy. But the funniest, most memorable story about vaginas, emotions, and orgasms came from a fellow author who heard about my work on this book and volunteered to share insights. So, from author and speaker Lori Ann King (*Come Back Strong: Balanced Wellness After Surgical Menopause*), here is the story of her menopausal re-entry into intimacy with her husband, Jim.

> Surgery at age 43 sent me into sudden surgical menopause. Intercourse was off the table for six weeks. I sat in the doctor's office at my six-week checkup, discussing reentry into the world of sex. My husband, Jim, and the doctor joked a bit as they sang a line of Madonna's "Like a Virgin." To warn you and to be frank, that's not quite accurate.
>
> My first time after surgery felt like my vagina had shortened, shrunk, and dried up. While there is controversy over whether the vagina shrinks due to surgery, the reality is that our vaginas are resilient. They can, after all, bounce back after childbirth. Or so they tell me. They can bounce back after a full hysterectomy as well.
>
> I found that the more relaxed I was, the less pain I had. I made sure I always had lubricant on hand and I used it early on to give my body all

the help it required. This became a fun time of exploration as together Jim and I learned what got my juices flowing. Literally.

Sex and intimacy are not only physical. They are emotional. This is where desire comes in, otherwise known as libido. I once heard that when a man and woman fight, the woman needs to resolve the issue before she has sex. A man needs to have sex before he can resolve the issue. I say sex has a similar effect as exercise: If you ask me how my day was before a workout, you'll get a very different response than you will if you wait to ask me after.

When I complained about a low libido, my doctor prescribed bioidentical testosterone. I fully expected Bioidentical Hormone Replacement Therapy (BHRT) to fix this, however, I did not notice significant improvement.

I kept an open mind and I recognized that sex brings a level of intimacy, communication, and relaxation to my marriage. I enjoy this closeness with Jim. So, I changed my expectations about BHRT and my mind about my libido. I took responsibility for my thoughts and feelings about my physical and sexual relationship. I embraced spontaneity as a grateful participant. I found that this approach always has a beautiful result: Orgasms bring joy, relaxation, and a deeper connection.

They also make me forget about my symptoms. And the laundry, the dishes, and anything on my chore list. Heck, sometimes I even forget my name.[2]

ENDING VAGINAL DRYNESS

Alyssa Dweck is a practicing gynecologist in Westchester County and maintains a popular blog focused on women's health issues. She put vaginal dryness in perspective in this way:

> The thing to note about hot flashes is that eventually they go away. The one thing about vaginal dryness and the changes in the vagina is that it's progressive and it will not get better by itself—ever. You have to manage it, especially if you want to maintain a sexual life, or just want to be free of discomfort caused by lack of estrogen. Left unaddressed, it can get worse as the years go on.[3]

We have four ways to fight vaginal dryness, one of which was explored in chapter 3 in the discussion of systemic hormone therapy. In addition, many lubricants, moisturizers, and energy-based devices have been proven effective in treating vaginal atrophy.

The two big questions dominating the fight to end vaginal dryness are: "What works?" and "What works *and* is good for my health—or at least won't hurt it?" The first question can be answered with the names of household pantry items, but the question worth answering is obviously the second one.

Lubes

Carol Queen, who holds a doctorate in sexology and is an executive with the women-founded Good Vibrations sex toy store in San Francisco, contributed many insights to the second half of this book. One of them is that there is no lube that is perfect for everyone. Just as we all have slightly different diets that work for us in terms of sustaining a sense of well-being, we can (and will) have different choices in lubricants.

Lubricants—commonly called lubes—can be oil-based, water-based, and silicone-based. In ranking cost, from lowest to highest, that's generally the order, although there are a number of variables that can affect cost. A number of variables can also affect how well the product works for intercourse versus toys, and whether you can be assured you have protected your health.

Now that you've seen the options, here's the recommendation: **Generally, avoid oil-based lubes.** The health risks should be a deterrent for frequent lube users. Consider what might happen before grabbing that extra virgin olive oil—or even the coconut oil—from the cabinet:

- Oils can clog your pores and clogged pores can lead to infection. Consider how it feels to put oil on your face: You may have an immediate sensation of smoothness and suppleness, but at some point, you want to wash it off so that your pores can breathe.
- If you are prone to yeast infections, then even organic extra virgin coconut oil is a bad option for lubrication. Coconut oil has the poten-

tial to upset the pH balance in the vaginal space, and the result could be a yeast infection.

- Exploring that point just a bit further, oils that are part of our food also serve as food for little critters like yeast.
- You can be putting pesticides into your body by using oil from your pantry unless it is a certified organic oil. Residues of pesticides used to ward off pests and weeds have been shown to contaminate the oil produced from the affected plants.[4]
- Oils can become rancid, and that might happen on your skin or in the bottle.
- Oils can be processed from sources that cause an allergic reaction for some people, such as beans or nuts. You may not be allergic to them, but what about your partner, who suddenly finds himself in close contact with peanut oil? Explain that to the emergency room doctor.

If, after all these warnings, you still want the pleasure, convenience, and cost-effectiveness associated with an oil-based lubricant, just make choices based on what's healthy for you.

- Choose high-quality virgin, unrefined coconut oil. It shouldn't cause the irritation or dryness associated with the partially hydrogenated and refined versions of the oil. Read the label: It should say "100% organic virgin coconut oil." Nothing else.
- A good nut oil is almond, which is less susceptible to becoming rancid than something like olive oil. Again, make sure it is organic and purified. And take the time to ask your partner if he or she has a nut allergy.

Turning to **water-based lubes**, many deliver the same slippery satisfaction as oils. There are different upsides and downsides associated with these other types of lubes, however. Here are a few overarching cautions:

- Some products become stickier than others during use. Read the label and see if words like "never sticky" or "does not leave a sticky residue" appear on the label. Marketing copy is no guarantee of result, but it can give you some idea of what to expect.

- Expect to have to reapply them during your sexual experience. Water-based lubes are designed to be compatible with skin, but because of that, there will be some absorption.
- The vagina is a mucous membrane, like the inside of the mouth. As such, it absorbs fluids at a higher rate than skin. The reason for listing chemicals in Table 6.1 is so you can get a better sense of which ones are naturally occurring, potentially irritating, considered benign, and so on. If you irrigate the vagina and/or surrounding areas with a lubricant—by throwing off the pH balance, for example—you run the risk of painful inflammation and infection. Hence the next caution.
- At any sign of itching or burning, stop using the lubricant. Throw it away. Never give it another try.

Based on ingredient information available at the time the book was developed, Table 6.1 provides a sampling of products that are water-based. They were selected on the basis of the different formulas they use. The aim is to provide you with information about products and ingredients to which many women are exposed. Please keep in mind that this is not (by far!) a comprehensive list, nor does it inherently contain any judgments about the efficacy of these products.

This table is meant primarily to show the order of ingredients, as well as why those ingredients are contained in a lubricant. Comments illuminate how those ingredients may relate to function and quality.

Do not shy away from the chemistry. Too many of the decisions that women make about skin care and other products are based on getting a good effect or liking the way they feel, even though they contain ingredients that might cause irritation or health issues over time. Others have bizarre-sounding ingredients that are perfectly safe, are already part of the human body, or are actually good for us. The substances mentioned in the table are some that you will see again and again on labels of products you use regularly. Simply take heed: Know why they are included in the formula and why you might either want to switch products or have a greater comfort level with those products.

In doing the research for this book, and probing into what lubes on the shelves contained, I finally found answers to why physical therapists, doctors, friends, and other women I interviewed liked and trusted certain water-based products and why other products might best be avoided. Note: Cost is not always the best criterion for judging ingredients, although huge cost differences should get your eyes focused on ingredients rather than compelling marketing copy.

It is also important to point out that frequency of use can make a huge difference in which product you ultimately choose. Infrequent use of a lube would likely mean you could use anything that enhances comfort and pleasure. In contrast, frequent use demands that you look very closely at ingredients and are not prone to the urinary tract infections or other problems that can arise from exposing yourself to the sugar-alcohol ingredients, for example. In an online survey I conducted of women over forty-five years, nearly one out of five said she used a lube either "regularly" or "usually." I am hoping women in that group look closely at this table and learn what may enhance their health and intimate experience rather than ultimately undermine them. And even the 22 percent who said they used a lube "sometimes" would benefit from doing comparison shopping using the information in the table. As for the slightly more than 40 percent who said they never used lube, I have only one caution: Vaginal atrophy can cause horrible urinary problems and make any gynecologic exam potentially painful. Please don't skip those exams just because you are menopausal or postmenopausal, and please use something to mitigate the thinning and drying of your vaginal walls due to the reduction in your estrogen production.

Silicone-based lubes have comfort advantages, but they will damage silicone toys, some of which are quite expensive due to their simulation of the feeling of skin. A main advantage of silicone-based lubes is that they are hypoallergenic, so the cautions for women about urinary tract infections that are associated with water-based lubes do not apply here.

Because they are not water-based, these lubricants will not dry up or evaporate during use. In that sense, they are similar in comfort to oil-based lubes. They will also not be absorbed into the body and are a better choice if used while having fun in a hot tub or your backyard swimming pool, for example.

Now think about it: If the lube has staying power in a pool, it will have staying power on your sheets and clothing. And your vagina. Use it sparingly and clean up afterward.

Table 6.1. A Sampling of Water-Based Vaginal Lubricants

Water-Based Product	Ingredients	Comments/Purpose in Formula
K-Y Water-Based Personal Lubricant; comparable to Wal-Mart Equate brand Lubricating Jelly	Purified water, glycerin, hydroxyethylcellulose, chlorhexidine gluconate, methylparaben, gluconolactone, sodium hydroxide	Glycerin, or glycerol, is a humectant and therefore attracts water; it helps to pull water to the wall of the vagina. It's a sugar, though, so anyone prone to yeast infections should be cautious of this ingredient in lubes. Read on to see the very last ingredient added to the formula, which theoretically would work to mitigate the risk of yeast infections. Hydroxyethylcellulose is derived from cellulose, a key structural component in green plants; it's water soluble and primarily used as a thickening agent. Chlorhexidine gluconate is a disinfectant and antiseptic. Methylparaben is a preservative. Gluconolactone is a natural substance with skin-conditioning properties. Sodium hydroxide, commonly called lye, is a very alkaline ingredient; its function in a lube is to control the pH of a product. See the note on coconut oil to understand the significance of that if you are prone to yeast infections.
Slippery Stuff	Deionized water, polyoxyethylene, sodium-carbomer, phenoxyethanol, ethylhexylglycerin	Deionized water is purified, but purified water may be distilled rather than deionized. The salient point is that both have impurities removed. Polyoxyethylene is a surfactant, meaning it lowers surface tension between two liquids, and an emulsifier, so it stabilizes the mixture. Sodium-carbomer is a thickener. Phenoxyethanol is a preservative. Ethylhexylglycerin is a skin conditioner.
		This product is one of many promoted as a "glycerin-free formula," which is relevant to women prone to urinary tract infections and yeast infections, as noted in the text.

Isabel Fay

Purified water, propanediol, citric acid, hydroxyethylcellulose, hydroxypropyl methylcellulose, potassium sorbate, sodium benzoate, xanthan gum

Propanediol aids skin conditioning by promoting the absorption of ingredients into skin. Citric acid is a natural ingredient found in a lot of fruits and juices, but in skin care it's used to adjust acidity. Referring again to the discussions of pH balance, acidity and alkalinity are important in the discussion of lubricants. The function and value of hydroxyethylcellulose was covered previously. Similarly, hydroxypropyl methylcellulose is a thickener, stabilizer, and lubricating substance; it tends to get thicker at higher temperatures—and that should not necessarily be construed as a negative in this context. Potassium sorbate is a preservative and considered a paraben alternative, meaning that it's a natural way to squelch the growth of microorganisms that would spoil the product. Sodium benzoate is another preservative—a salt—that is found naturally in cranberries, plums, apples, and other fruits. Xanthan gum sounds like something awful, but it's something that has the capacity to hold water and improve shelf life, so despite its unnatural sounding name, it's considered benign.

Genneve Intimate Moisture

Water, glyceryl polymethacrylate, glycerin, sorbitol, propylene glycol, panthenol, sodium hyaluronate, sodium PCA, PEG-90M, carbomer, sodium hydroxide, diazolidinyl urea, disodium EDTA

Polymethacrylate is used to enhance the texture and application of the product. Like glycerin, sorbitol is a sugar-like alcohol used to prevent moisture loss. The caution has already been made about sugar-like alcohols and women prone to yeast infections, but in this case, the interesting addition is that the Genneve product tastes good; a subtle, pleasant sweetness may be attributable to the sorbitol. Propylene glycol is a plant-based humectant,

(continued)

Table 6.1. *(Continued)*

Water-Based Product	Ingredients	Comments/Purpose in Formula
		and it's similar to glycerin in some key ways. Panthenol is a vitamin B5 derivative that has a lubricating and hydrating effect. Sodium hyaluronate helps restore moisture and prevent friction so common uses are in treatment of joint pain and dry eyes. (See the discussion of hyaluronic acid in the section on moisturizers.) Sodium PCA occurs in human skin and has a moisturizing effect. PEG-90M is not the name of a science fiction movie; it stands for polyethylene glycol, and there are many variations, with 90M being a compound used in some cosmetics as a penetration enhancer. Carbomer is made from acrylic acid, and it's a powder often added to makeup, skin care products, and even toothpaste as a thickener. Again, sodium hydroxide is all about balancing pH, covered in the first entry. Diazolidinyl urea is a preservative. Disodium EDTA is another preservative, but it's also considered a penetration enhancer.
Sliquid H20 (The company also offers a silicon-based lube called Sliquid Silver)	Purified water, plant cellulose, cyamopsis, potassium sorbate, citric acid	Cyamopsis is the one item in the list that may be unfamiliar. It's also known as guar gum and is a commonly used thickener.

Non-Estrogen Moisturizers

We are generally more familiar with vaginal lubricants than moisturizers, mostly because they are considered topical formulas. In contrast, when a product is intended to provide a benefit when introduced inside the body, to some degree, there is involvement of the Food and Drug Administration (FDA) in the United States, the European Medicines Agency, the Pharmaceutical and Medical Devices Agency in Japan, and so on. These are products that are used on an ongoing basis to ease painful intercourse, meaning that they are designed to address persistent issues of vaginal dryness in a way that allows for spontaneous sexual activity. A moisturizer is designed to replenish vaginal moisture; it involves a continuing commitment.

Unlike lubricants, moisturizers are likely to be associated with studies published in medical journals. For example, a study published in the *New England Journal of Medicine* in 2006 stated:

> In a randomized trial, a polycarbophil-based vaginal moisturizer available over the counter (Replens) provided relief of vaginal symptoms that was equivalent to that of vaginal estrogen and also lowered vaginal pH.[5]

Polycarbophil is an "acidic, inert, bioadhesive polymer that allows the product to attach to the walls of the vagina," according to *Consumer Health Digest*,[6] which gave Replens a positive rating. The only caution is one that would apply to any product, that is, check the ingredient list to make sure you don't have an allergy to anything in the formula such as mineral oil or hydrogenated palm oil glyceride. K-Y Liquibeads is another product with a silicon-based polymer featured in its formula. With this product, the usual warning about glycerin and its link to yeast infections would apply. Replens requires an applicator; K-Y Liquibeads are ovules.

Revaree is a product introduced in mid-2018 to address vaginal dryness and in some fundamental ways differs from others that preceded it in the marketplace. Like the products mentioned previously, it is non-hormonal and intended to hydrate vaginal tissues, rather than just lubricate them. A vaginal insert, or vaginal suppository, is introduced into the vagina three or four times a week, depending on need. The ingredients per vaginal insert are simple and listed as hyaluronic acid sodium salt 5 mg and semi-synthetic glycerides. The latter is an excipient for suppositories, meaning that it's an inactive substance serving as the delivery mechanism for an active ingredient.

As is the case with certain creams that have been used in the vaginal area, hyaluronic acid is the superstar. It's a natural substance found in the body's connective, neural, and epithelial tissues (skin, for example, as well as the outer surfaces of organs and blood vessels), with the highest concentrations in the eyes and joints.

Hyaluronic acid is featured in a number of products aiding pain relief, promoting healing, and providing rejuvenation effects for various parts of the body. Since the 1990s, it's been a popular ingredient in anti-aging, dermatologic products; some plastic surgeons also use it as a lip filler. In the prior decade, it started being used extensively during certain types of eye surgeries as well as in orthopedics. As far back as the 1960s, researchers determined that hyaluronic acid has an important role in cell metabolism and in facilitating tissue repair, so its first medical uses were treating skin lesions.

JDS Therapeutics was permitted to bring Revaree to market after a number of clinical trials, which were inherent in the process of securing FDA clearance as a medical device. Lubricants intended for external use do not have to meet requirements that apply to medical devices. There was also a precedent for using hyaluronic acid for treatment of vaginal dryness, so the FDA had considered that in providing the clearance.[7]

Prior to the product coming to market, a team of researchers from Shiraz University of Medical Science in Iran conducted a study, published in 2016, involving menopausal women and the effect of hyaluronic cream versus conjugated estrogen on their vaginal atrophy, or dryness. The results made hyaluronic acid-based product look like a more promising remedy for dryness than the estrogen-containing cream they used (Premarin). One of the unexpected findings was that urinary incontinence, as well as dryness, showed improvement in the group using the hyaluronic acid.

> According to the results of the present study, hyaluronic acid and conjugated estrogen improved the symptoms of vaginal atrophy. But hyaluronic acid was more effective and this drug is suggested for those who do not want to or cannot take local hormone treatment.[8]

The issue of who can and who cannot take local hormone treatment is an important one. The safety information and indications material for Premarin cream states:

Using estrogen-alone may increase your chance of getting cancer of the uterus (womb). Report any unusual vaginal bleeding right away while you are using Premarin (conjugated estrogens) Vaginal Cream. Vaginal bleeding after menopause may be a warning sign of cancer of the uterus (womb). Your healthcare provider should check any unusual vaginal bleeding to find out the cause.[9]

Those of us who used Premarin cream and were subsequently diagnosed with uterine cancer urge every woman to take this warning seriously. Some of us are simply not good candidates for this product and should pursue non-hormonal alternatives such as those covered in this section. Doctors and physician assistants need to read the cautions before they prescribe.

Treatments with Energy-Based Devices

Is there really a "permanent" fix for the vaginal and vulvar deterioration associated with menopause? That's the hype associated with laser and radiofrequency treatments. Given that these treatments have long been used within dermatology and plastic surgery to stimulate the production of new collagen and elastic fibers, using them to restore vaginal tissue was just a logical next step. Particularly menopausal women who have had breast or endometrial cancer should investigate energy-based treatment as they are not considered good candidates for estrogen therapy.

A distinct downside of the energy device treatments for most women is the cost. Fees range from a low of one thousand dollars for certain physicians providing laser treatments up to thirty-five hundred dollars for some of the radiofrequency treatments. These fees would cover the first series of treatments with follow-ups costing far less. And even though these treatments address chronic issues that many women would say cause pain and affect their quality of life, laser and radiofrequency treatments are currently not covered by insurance—at least, not completely. In the case of severe pelvic prolapse (extreme weakness in muscles supporting the uterus, bladder, and rectum) or stress urinary incontinence, some insurance companies might provide a partial reimbursement, but you can expect your doctor to want full payment when services are rendered.

Without any, or much, help from insurance, women on a tight budget would put this option low on the list for now. For this reason, clusters of providers are generally found in relatively high-wealth areas.

The costs of hormone therapy, or even some non-hormonal therapies, can add up. The big financial differences, of course, are that hormone therapy can be covered by insurance and the costs are generally spread over time.

Table 6.2 provides an overview of the two types of energy-based devices now in use to aid internal and external vaginal rejuvenation.

Lasers

Vaginal laser therapy—especially FemiLift and IntimaLase—got a big boost in visibility from a 2016 article in *Glamour Magazine*. Following Khloe Kardashian's remark during an episode of the television reality series *Kocktails with Khloe* that her sisters who had given birth used a "vagina lasering thing to tighten,"[10] *Glamour* mentioned the two devices in "Yup, Laser Vaginal Tightening Is a Thing. Here's What It's All About."

Laser devices also have earned serious attention from the medical community. IntimaLase and Petit Lady—both lasers emitting infrared light—received positive reviews after clinical trials. The conclusion was that the Er:YAG laser treatment "led to significant decrease in both vaginal dryness and dyspareunia as well as significant improvement of urinary incontinence."[11]

In 2014, after several outcome studies, the MonaLisa Touch vaginal laser treatment received approval from the FDA for gynecologic use. It had been approved for such use in Europe in 2008. It is one of several fractionated carbon dioxide lasers—light transmitted through carbon dioxide—which is exactly the kind of lasers used by plastic surgeons and dermatologists to treat facial wrinkles. The big difference is that the physicians who initially thought of using it for vaginal rejuvenation turned down the intensity. A very important outcome of the initial work was evidence that use of the laser mitigated more than one effect of estrogen deprivation, namely, the therapy addressed both vaginal/vulvar deterioration and problems of incontinence. Six scientific publications confirm the effectiveness and safety of this device.[12]

Rebecca Dunsmoor-Su, a physician specializing in menopause and currently one of only two gynecologists in the Seattle area with the

Table 6.2. Laser and Radiofrequency-Based Devices for Vaginal Rejuvenation

Laser-Based Devices		Number of Treatments (T)
FemiLift Alma Lasers	Fractional carbon dioxide laser	Three treatments at four- to six-week intervals
MonaLisa Touch, Cynosure	Fractional carbon dioxide laser	Three treatments at six-week intervals
IntimaLase, Fotona	Er:YAG (an infrared light laser)	Two treatments at eight-week intervals
Petit Lady, Lutronic	Er:YAG	Three treatments at two-week intervals
Radiofrequency-Based Devices		
ThermiVa, ThermiAesthetics	Temperature-controlled radiofrequency	Three treatments at four- to six-week intervals
ReVive, Viora	Bipolar radiofrequency	Four to six treatments at two- to three-week intervals
Venus Fiore, VenusConcept	Multipolar-radiofrequency with pulsed electromagnetic field	Three treatments at one-week intervals
Viveve System, Viveve Medical	Patented radiofrequency	One treatment
Protégé Intima, BTL Aesthetics	Focused radiofrequency	Two to four treatments every two to three weeks
Pelleve, Ellman International	Monopolar radiofrequency	Three treatments at two- to three-week intervals

credentials to use the MonaLisa Touch, offers this explanation of how the therapy works:

> The laser makes tiny microinjuries in the vaginal tissue and the vulva, because we do an external treatment as well. Those microinjuries then cause a healing reaction. The body heals those tissues, and in the process of healing those tissues, the body resets to what it sees as normal. And what it sees as normal is pre-menopausal tissue. So you get collagen ingrowth and you get vascular ingrowth and you get hydration of the tissues. All of that means that the tissues become more structurally sound and thicker.[13]

Results have been a return of elasticity, premenopausal levels of hydration, and thicker more resilient tissue—all of which contribute to both vaginal and vulvar health and an elimination of sexual discomfort. Whether or not greater sexual pleasure is part of the package is not a matter for the doctor, but a matter of your relationship, of course.

One of the most recent studies undertaken about the efficacy of the MonaLisa laser is sponsored by the Michigan Institution of Women's Health and was announced in November 2017.[14] The aim of the study is to determine the effect of this particular device on a serious problem that plagues many women who are in menopause or postmenopausal, namely genitourinary syndrome (GSM). All of the elements of GSM have been mentioned previously in this book, but here they are again in one place, as described by the study summary:

> progressive worsening of the vaginal and vulvar anatomy with symptoms of vulvar itching or pain during intercourse, vaginal dryness, urinary urgency and frequency and frequent bladder infections. It could ultimately lead to vaginal bleeding, petechial hemorrhages, vaginal narrowing or stenosis and hypertonicity of the pelvic muscles due to anticipation of coital pain. The hypertonicity by itself can cause pelvic pressure or pain. Thus, GSM is a chronic progressive disease state that if left untreated could have dire vaginal and urogynecological consequences.[15]

I feel it's important to clarify the description of GSM as a "disease state" because menopause itself is not a disease, yet recognizing some of the outcomes of estrogen depletion as "disease states" has some value—not the least of which is in getting insurance companies to cover the costs of therapy. The message is: This is a condition that undermines health, and it needs to be addressed.

The reason the study was designed is specifically because of the observed and clinically documented benefits described by Dunsmoor-Su, that is, the ability of the laser treatment to stimulate the synthesis of collagen "and stratification of the vaginal epithelium with improvement of the vaginal pH and moisturization of the vaginal tissue due to increased blood flow."[16]

The typical treatment schedule is three sessions of laser spaced at six weeks apart, with each treatment lasting only about five minutes. For most women, that is sufficient for the year. They would come back annually for a checkup and one-time session. In the vagina, the laser feels like a buzzing or humming, but due to the many nerve endings in the vulva—there are more than eight thousand nerve endings in the clitoris—a numbing ointment is used prior to treatment.

Dunsmoor-Su treated 120 women in the two-year period of 2016 to 2018 after she received her training with the device. In determining whether the procedure was successful, she asks her patients two questions, "Is it better than it was before?" and "Did you get the result you wanted?" Nearly 100 percent of the women say their vaginal and vulva condition is better than before. She puts the success rate with the second question at 85 percent. The primary changes inherent in that response are no painful intercourse, feeling well hydrated, and no itching and burning.

A main determinant of success is how long the woman has been in menopause. Physicians using the laser are trying to stimulate tissues that have been dormant for a while. As Dunsmoor-Su explains, "Trying to wake up tissue that has been asleep for twenty years is harder than trying to wake up tissue that has been asleep for five years."[17]

Expectations that any laser device delivers a miracle cure are not realistic—at least not for all women. Much of the dramatic success depends on a women's age and experience going into the process. If, for example, a woman has been having painful intercourse for close to ten years, the treatment can make the tissues better; however, that alone won't put her sex life back on track immediately. The fact that she has been having intercourse despite the discomfort means that she might have a pelvic floor spasm whenever she has attempted intercourse; it's a natural, protective response to pain. Once the tissues are better, the next step is to find a physical therapist who can treat the pelvic floor issues so the woman can relax and enjoy intercourse again.

Dunsmoor-Su also notes that certain conditions make getting the desired result much more challenging than usual. Her experience is anecdotal, but worth noting; hopefully, future studies will illuminate the importance of these conditions in getting a good result. One challenge relates to women on aromatase inhibitors, which would be taken by postmenopausal women as part of treatment for breast cancer. Aromatase is an enzyme that synthesizes estrogen, the hormone that feeds breast cancer tumors. Women on aromatase inhibitors can still get a good result with treatment, but it may take more sessions.

Women who have lichen sclerosus, an autoimmune attack on the vulva that causes a thinning of the tissues, fissuring, itching, and burning, also need more frequent treatments than usual.

A third category of patient that may not respond as well to the laser therapy is women who have had radiation in the pelvic area. It may not always be possible to rejuvenate tissues exposed to radiation. Vaginal brachytherapy is a post-surgical, and possibly also a post-chemotherapy, treatment for endometrial cancer. It involves placing a source of radiation into a cylinder and inserting it into the vagina, generally just for a few minutes at a time. The upper part of the vagina is always treated because if there were any stray cancer cells remaining after the hysterectomy, this is where they would probably be. The radiation mainly affects the area of the vagina in contact with the cylinder, which explains why the tissues in the area can be permanently damaged and unresponsive to laser treatment. The laser will not make anything worse, but it may not make it better. That said, Dunsmoor-Su said that the three women she has treated who have had radiation did get good results, principally in the vulvar area, which is left out of the radiation field.

As a final note, despite the tissue resilience and hydration improvement that should come with the laser treatment, continued use of lubes is always a good idea.

Radiofrequency Devices

Refer to Table 6.2 to see the different ways the six radiofrequency devices are described. Marketing material might lead you to believe one has some kind of revolutionary advantage over the other; however, let's focus on what they have in common. Just like lasers, radiofrequency devices are meant to stimulate the production of new collagen and elastic fibers. They are also non-surgical, involve a short office visit, and do not require anesthesia.

COOLING HOT FLASHES AND NIGHT SWEATS

What woman wants to have hot sex when she feels like her body is already on fire? Or roll over and cuddle her partner when the sheets are drenched in sweat?

Chapter 3 covered the hormone-based, systemic therapies used to manage vasomotor symptoms of menopause, that is night sweats, hot flashes, and flushes. With the focus on non-hormonal treatments here, we will explore the first—and as of this writing, the only—FDA-approved non-hormonal medication as well as non-hormonal, non-medicine approaches that work well for some women. The so-called natural remedies that are taken orally are composed of bioidenticals and received coverage in chapter 3.

The Antidepressant

In July 2013, the FDA approved Brisdelle, made by Noven Pharmaceuticals, as a treatment for vasomotor symptoms of menopause. The key ingredient is an antidepressant, a selective serotonin reuptake inhibitor, sold under the brand names of Paxil and Pexeva. Taken once a day at bedtime, Brisdelle is convenient. But despite study results showing a statistically significant reduction in the frequency and severity of symptoms compared to a placebo, the drug has downsides. It carries with it the same warnings that the other antidepressants carry.

The Brisdelle website warns about possible suicidal thoughts and depression. It's ironic that antidepressants can cause depression, but studies indicate that it does happen—and women who had previously been on antidepressants are especially vulnerable. One study published in 2011 in *Frontiers of Psychology* found that people diagnosed with depression who had been antidepressant users had about a 42 percent chance of a relapse versus the 25 percent chance for patients with depression who never took the drugs.[18]

Another serious health consequence that can surface with use of the drug is serotonin syndrome, which the site says may include:

> Nervousness, hallucinations, coma, or other changes in mental status; coordination problems or small movements of the muscles that you cannot control; racing heartbeat, high or low blood pressure; sweating or fever; nausea, vomiting, or diarrhea; muscle rigidity; dizziness; flushing; tremors; seizures.[19]

In addition, women being treated for breast cancer with tamoxifen may find that Brisdelle doesn't work as well for them as it does for others because of the drug interaction. Another unfavorable drug interaction occurs when Brisdelle and blood thinners, or even ibuprofen or aspirin, are taken at the same time.

Noven has to issue these warnings, as do any companies with FDA reviewed and certified products—and they are not just fine print that can be ignored. As discussions of Premarin indicated, a woman relying on a treatment that can pose serious health risks should not assume that a doctor's recommendation on using it means those warnings are irrelevant.

Herbs and Eats

The North American Menopause Society (www.menopause.org) posed a provocative question: "Do Mother Nature's Treatments Help Hot Flashes?"[20] After reviewing countless claims, I would say their analyses of herbal benefits are reliable based on current data. Following is an analysis of the value of herbal treatments based on that data:

- Black cohosh: Contrary to what people in the medical/health community thought originally, this herb does not act like estrogen. That's good news for women looking for non-hormonal relief from hot flashes, but the less-than-good news is that studies do not confirm it helps hot flashes. The study results are mixed, and the affirmations of its value are largely anecdotal.
- Red clover: Again, the positive stories about its ability to relieve hot flashes are anecdotal, so anyone with a science-based orientation would wonder if there is simply a placebo effect happening. Five controlled studies of red clover extract have indicated no conclusive evidence that it has any ability to reduce hot flashes.[21]

- Dong quai: Called the "female ginseng" because of its supposed balancing effect in the body, this herb has been made into tea and capsules, and it has been put on an altar by people who swear by its reliable use in Chinese medicine for more than a thousand years. It is a member of the celery family that can affect nerve endings that release and are stimulated by serotonin. (Please go back to the discussion on antidepressants to read how serotonins and hot flashes might be connected.) Chinese medicine practitioners have long argued that the value of dong quai may be misunderstood because the preparations commonly available are not what *they* use—and a major study indicated they are probably right. The 2013 study indicated inconclusive results about the efficacy of dong quai in helping mitigate menopausal symptoms because of the need for "well-defined extracts" to delineate the true potential of the herb.[22] If you have a Chinese medicine practitioner you trust, you may have different results from women relying on the multiple commercial sources of the herb extract.
- Ginseng: A hot ginseng tea at bedtime might help with sleep issues, and a few cups during the day might mitigate mood swings. Don't rely on it for any relief of hot flashes or night sweats, though.
- Evening primrose oil: The hype has been that it helps with hot flashes, but the contraindications for use after randomized studies are so alarming that this seems like something to stay away from.

The discussion of bioidenticals in chapter 3 referenced how plant sources of estrogen make their way into compounds called "natural" even though the sources are processed in a lab. But then, there is the possibility of having the source be natural by eating part or all of the actual plants.

Soybeans, chickpeas, and lentils are especially good sources of isoflavones, which are phytoestrogens, that is, plant sources of estrogen. You'll never get the same infusion of estrogen from eating tofu and hummus as you will from hormone therapy, but you may get mild relief from hot flashes and other symptoms.

The claim that isoflavones can help relieve menopause symptoms is no longer just anecdotal, or something shaping the script of a few scenes in *Sex and the City 2*. A 2017 study published in the *Journal of Clinical & Diagnostic Research* affirmed that ingesting one hundred milligrams per day of soy isoflavones over a twelve-week period showed measurable improvement in their hot flashes.[23] You could get that one hundred-milligram daily dose of soy isoflavones in capsule form, or just eat the right amount of soy. A cup of boiled soybeans gives you nearly one hundred milligrams and so does about two cups of tofu.

Women with a genetic predisposition to breast cancer or who have survived breast cancer have been warned against dietary isoflavones, but the latest research shows that might be an overreaction. While there is a link between estrogen and breast cancer risk, it isn't clear that dietary sources of phytoestrogens contribute to the risk. In fact, the team conducting a 2017 study published in *Medicines* concluded that dietary isoflavones "possess both antiestrogenic and estrogenic effects on breast cancer cells."[24] In other words, they could have both a protective and a risk-increasing effect.

Acupuncture and More

> Science is on your side with acupuncture. Let's cut to the good news immediately: The severity of hot flushes was found to be significantly decreased after treatment in the acupuncture group. . . . Acupuncture was effective in reducing menopausal complaints when compared to sham acupuncture and can be considered as an alternative therapy in the treatment of menopausal symptoms.[25]

What you need to know about this is that hot flashes and night sweats can be countered with acupuncture in many cases; in fact, many women reported a reduction in symptoms of almost half.[26] My personal experience of acupuncture suggests that a good practitioner delivers symptom relief that is painless and affordable. Be patient, though: Give the treatments three or four weeks to make a noticeable difference.

How does sticking needles into skin potentially reduce major vasomotor menopause symptoms so significantly?

Acupuncture needles first received FDA approval in 1996 as medical devices. With proper use, they activate the body's own self-healing mechanisms. In fact, that is the premise of the healing value of acupuncture: It's alerting the body what it can be doing for itself.

Women who cannot do hormone therapy and/or have an authentic orientation toward natural, non-drug therapies should consider acupuncture to reduce their hot flashes and night sweats. Interestingly, though, the reason *exactly* why it works is a little fuzzy.

One theory is that acupuncture stimulates the release of endorphins, which are hormones that reduce pain and cause a sense of well-being. Another possibility, and a corollary to the other one, is that acupuncture affects the hypothalamus of the brain. This is an almond-sized part of the brain that controls certain metabolic processes in the body, including body temperature and hormone production. So a laywoman's interpretation of this is that acupuncture can relieve pain, make you feel good, and affect your personal thermostat.

Four other techniques in this category are worth considering in mitigating vasomotor symptoms of menopause: meditation, visualization, exercise, use of ice, and massage. Most likely, these will not be primary means of dealing with moderate to severe symptoms; however, they may be very useful as adjunct therapies.

- Meditation: Hot flashes are notorious for triggering anxiety. Meditation techniques help you focus on breathing that relaxes the mind and body. Used in conjunction with other therapies, this could help you sleep better and have confidence that everything else you're doing is worth the effort.
- Visualization: Let me tell you a story about how powerful visualization really is. It may seem a little one-off, but that is precisely what makes it memorable and therefore useful. I hope it will inspire you to realize that your imagination, your dreaming, can have tremendous power over the events in your life—your sense of well-being, your possibilities for intimacy, and so much more. Brian Boitano won a gold medal in figure skating at the 1988 Olympics in Calgary. He had a coach, who was also one of my mindfulness coaches, in training the "inner body" to support the training of the "outer body." Brian was adept at using techniques that many athletes, as well as non-athletes seeking performance improvement, have now adopted to some degree, and one of them is visualization, which may be described as "sensualization" when multiple senses are involved. Brian told me this story about his win in Calgary and how visualization offered him both strength and delightful surprises:

"The Star-Spangled Banner" was playing and I said to myself, "This tempo is too fast." My nightly visualizations for about a year had been complete up until that moment—*exactly* as I'd visualized everything. The jumping, the way the audience responded, the way I responded to the audience. First I did this, then I cried, then I laughed—all that was visualized. When it happened, it was like I was dreaming. It was surreal to me. Then I got up to the podium after winning the gold medal and the National Anthem started playing and I thought, "This isn't 'The Star-Spangled Banner' that I imagined. It's too fast!" I imagined "The Star-Spangled Banner" going, "Daaah, daaah, daaah, daaah, dah," but it started differently. The drums came in ad it was "dah, dah, dah, dah, dah, dah," and I thought, "This is not real! The tempo's wrong!" That's what made me realize it *was* real.[27]

More than any story I have ever heard, Brian's exemplifies the power of the mind in working *with* the body to produce amazing results. In a variety of life situations, including the exploration of intimacy, I have remembered this story and found it both inspiring and practical.

- Exercise: As noted in chapter 1, exercise appears to be an effective way to mitigate the number and intensity of hot flashes. Exercise prepares the body to manage the temperature changes much more efficiently, particularly reducing the amount of sweat generated during a hot flash.
- Ice: Use ice packs with protective coverings so you will not "burn" your skin and put them on your forehead and neck to get immediate relief. It's a quick fix without lasting results, but certainly worth adding to the mix of non-hormonal treatments.
- Massage: If you can afford the service and the time, an aromatherapy massage involving essential oils like rose and lavender can lower the intensity of your hot flashes, or even prevent them.

SLEEPING WITH INSOMNIA

For some women, restless sleep may be one of the first indications that they have entered a perimenopausal state. Along with the reduction in estrogen comes a drop in the level of progesterone, which is a sleep-promoting hormone. Add night sweats to that and a middle-aged woman may wonder if she'll ever get a good night's sleep again. Insomniacs tend to have a hard time falling asleep and/or wake up and cannot get back to sleep for a long time.

This can become a vicious cycle: Inability to sleep makes you less capable of managing symptoms of menopause and that leads to even less sleep. Your immune system, body temperature, and blood pressure will suffer. Your mood will suffer. You'll find yourself healing more slowly. And you really won't have much, if any, ability to enjoy any intimacy with your well-rested, energetic partner. The consequences of sleeplessness are so dramatic that Steven Lockley of Brigham and Women's Hospital in Boston believes that "sleep may be more essential to us than food."[28] With insomnia, you aren't just irritable and cognitively impaired, you are at risk of dying prematurely.

Joyce Walsleben writes for the National Sleep Foundation about menopause and insomnia, and her non-drug recommendations are straightforward. If followed while you are also using your therapies of choice to mitigate symptoms of menopause, they will help you improve your sleep:

- Make your room dark, quiet, and safe.
- Keep your room as cool as you can.
- Skip alcohol and tobacco.
- Keep a cloth in a bucket of ice near your bed so you can cool yourself quickly.[29]

Walsleben has another recommendation for perimenopausal women: a low-dose birth control pill. It has the potential to stabilize minor fluctuations in estrogen levels.

Several years ago, I did the non-medical research for a book on sleep I co-authored with the medical director of the Pennsylvania Hospital Sleep Disorders Center, Ronald L. Kotler. In *365 Ways to Get a Good Night's Sleep*, we devoted forty-five tips to non-drug and non-medical ways to address insomnia, including some already mentioned here, as ways to mitigate menopause symptoms, namely, acupuncture and massage therapy (including self-massage).

In our section on herbals, we cautioned against using valerian, even though it has the nickname "herbal Valium." Valerian can go both ways: ease you into sleep or stimulate you enough to keep you awake.[30] If you do decide to try it, be cautious and take less than the recommended dosage on the bottle. Also, note that melatonin is not a sleep aid. It helps to reset your body clock so, for example, it could enable you to go to bed at a reasonable time on the east coast after just traveling from the west coast of the United States. Finally, one safe option that is well understood is a cup of chamomile tea. You won't nod off immediately after drinking it, but you may feel a bit more relaxed than before.

To conclude, let's consider some happy news about sleeping that directly relates to sex. Dreams activate your body sexually whether you like it or not. Men get erections and women experience clitoral and vaginal engorgement.[31] Overcoming insomnia will be good for your sex life whether you are asleep or awake.

Chapter Seven

Finding a New Normal

Viewpoints

According to the Bible, humanity's downfall was all Eve's fault. She sought pleasure and that was the original sin:

> When the woman saw that the fruit of the tree was good for food and pleasing to the eye, and also desirable for gaining wisdom, she took some and ate it. She also gave some to her husband, who was with her, and he ate it. (Genesis 3:6)

God made it clear what they did was a mistake. What did Adam do? He put the blame on Eve: "The woman you put here with me—she gave me some fruit from the tree, and I ate it." (Genesis 3:12)

So within six verses of the first chapter in the Bible, we find out women who seek pleasure will be punished, men who want the same pleasure will forget everything and go for it, and anything bad that comes of it is the woman's fault. This is bad messaging for women, not to mention the fact that men don't deserve such a bad rap.

With that in mind, let's begin with the story of Janie. After many months of struggle, Janie had learned to effectively manage her menopause symptoms. Her husband Bruce hadn't wanted to "bother" her with requests for intimacy, so he just worked late and played golf with his buddies on the weekends. Even though Janie wasn't particularly interested in sex, she felt she ought to make an effort to reconnect with Bruce. She spent $1.19 on a package of fourteen little stickers that looked like lips and put them on his electric razor, computer keyboard, iPad cover, hairbrush, and other places where he would definitely notice them. Bruce did notice them and did not require any explanation; he knew they were an invitation. The most difficult part of reconnecting was not physical, however; it was that Janie didn't get as turned on as she'd hoped. How could she recover her libido? She tried Scream Cream, compounded to increase blood flow to the genitals and enhance orgasm. It did have an effect on sensation, but not desire.

Janie's story had lots of options for a happy ending, and they all came out of reorienting her point of view in relation to a very simple concept: pleasure.

THE PLEASURE PATH

Menopause is a socially accepted excuse for bouts of depression, erratic behavior, canceling plans, fat around the middle, health complaints, fatigue, and perfectly good excuses for not having sex. The alternative requires energy, commitment, and refusal to be a victim of Mother Nature—and it is an alternative filled with pleasure and joy.

In general, women have misconceptions about what pleasure should be like. We are socialized to associate pleasure with giving someone else pleasure. Movies, advertisements, and television shows hardly ever depict a sexual interaction as something in which the woman is the sole recipient of pleasure. Women are conditioned to think it's fine if they don't always have an orgasm; the important outcome is the man reaching a climax.

Women tend to be prevented from wanting and seeking pleasure. Only bad girls do that.

The socialization carries through menopause, with another layer of messaging affecting women and pleasure. After all those years of not being the center of pleasure activities, suddenly none of that matters because you're no longer going to want intimate relations anyway. And if you have sex, you're just trying to make the best of a bad situation; you feel a duty to your relationship to give your mate what he wants.

Menopause becomes a convenient excuse to *avoid* pleasure. Feeling sexually fulfilled is too much work and tinged with guilt.

Long before the onset of menopause, many women feel as though they don't have any other place to go—literally or figuratively—in terms of future pleasure. They are unaware of an alternative path because it's "dirty" to explore one. What would friends think? The people at their church? Their kids in high school?

Menopause presents the kind of choice that poet Robert Frost introduced in his 1916 classic *The Road Not Taken*. It begins "Two roads diverged in a yellow wood," and from there takes the reader into a consideration of which path to take as he continues on his journey. He chooses the road less traveled and concludes with "And that has made all the difference."

If you choose to take the road less traveled and discover, or rediscover, the pleasure in your intimate life, then this chapter can put some cairns on the trail to help you move forward and not get "lost."

Step 1: Decide that more pleasure is worth having in your life.

Instructors with The Welcomed Consensus would tell you that one of the most difficult areas to confront is your sensuality. Therefore, the first step is to decide "Yes. I am going to seek pleasure." Founded in 1992, The Welcomed Consensus teaches how to succeed in relationships with fun as a goal; their focus is female orgasm and its integral role in pleasurable living. Their instructors introduce women and men to viewpoints, tools, and techniques that help couples and singles recognize female pleasure as life-affirming, rather than a source of guilt, shame, or selfishness.

Your first step down the path to a more pleasurable life, therefore, is to decide you deserve and want pleasure. If that step seems emotionally jarring, try approaching the decision intellectually. You are going to become a "sensual researcher"—a Welcomed Consensus phrase—with your own body and mind as the focus of your research.

Step 2: Conduct sensual research.

Determine what feels good to you—on all levels.

A number of women I've spoken with get great satisfaction out of having their feet massaged. They feel comfortable admitting that, but won't explore how they feel when they, or a partner, moves up the legs and beyond. Figure out for yourself when and where on your body you prefer a light touch, heavy touch, or a good scratch. Do you prefer the feel of water to lotion, or lotion to oil? How does a cold drink on a hot day feel, and vice versa?

In the 1988 book *Safe Encounters*, Beverly Whipple, the sexologist who identified the G spot, and her co-author Gina Ogden offered readers an "extragenital matrix." It's a table to help women and men discover areas of sensual and sexual pleasure as well as what kind of nongenital touching makes a person feel good. The table, which is freely downloadable,[1] lists all the parts of the head and face, neck and torso, arms and hands, and legs and feet on the left. The table does not contain any reference to genitals, although there are plenty of other erogenous zones, or possible erogenous zones, on the list. Across the top are categories of touching by hand and mouth, and with other body parts. If you and your partner decided to explore together, you could choose a body part such as inner thighs and determine what felt best touching by hand (stroking, patting, rubbing, squeezing, pinching, spanking, other), by mouth (sucking, nuzzling, licking, fluttering, nipping, other), or with other parts (hugging, full body, hair massage, other). Self-exploration could include anything done by hand and, depending on the body part, anything done by mouth.

Using Whipple and Ogden's extragenital matrix is one way to begin your "work" as a sensual researcher. Exposure to a concept at the centerpiece of Masters and Johnson's therapeutic work could nudge you further into it.

Beginning in the 1960s, William Masters and Virginia Johnson essentially tried to turn men and women into sensual researchers through their work in sensate focus, the foundation of their sex therapy. In their paper "Sensate Focus: Clarifying the Masters and Johnson's Model," sexologists Linda Weiner and Constance Avery-Clark described the benefit of sensate focus as follows: "By mindfully being present to sensations in the moment, and refraining from forcing pleasure and arousal, clients can move toward the optimal intimacy they desire."[2] Both authors held research and clinical positions at the Masters & Johnson Institute in the mid- to late-1980s and had first-hand knowledge of how the therapy evolved over time.

In a clinical setting, the couple talks with a therapist about what they will be doing later in the privacy of their own home or hotel room. The sensate focus exercises are designed to heighten the level of trust and intimacy the two people feel for each other, with a crucial element being the cultivation of their ability to give and receive pleasure. It's not about orgasm; it's about pleasure, although certainly orgasm might result. It's important to note that sensate focus is an actual therapeutic program not to be confused with erotic touch, for example. Yet knowing something about it, even without going through it, can expand your thinking about the possibilities for sensual awareness.

In that it's directed toward pleasure, sensate focus therapy is somewhat philosophically in tune with the work of The Welcomed Consensus, although that is an organization of teachers, not therapists. They are a group of instructors who, rather than "cure" the sexual problems of troubled couples, offer winning viewpoints that are enlightening when applied in sexual situations. In addition, their work illuminates the value and virtue of *women* experiencing pleasure.

The University of Notre Dame provides a description of sensate focus exercise, and it is freely available online.[3] An opening statement captures why so many of us cannot seem to focus on our sensual natures in a way that fuels our enjoyment of life: We are distracted.

The opening of a video created by The Welcomed Consensus called "A Guide to Your Orgasm" features a sensual researcher named Rebecca demonstrating how to eliminate the distractions that undermine pleasure. These are simple actions similar to those taken by massage therapists who create a safe, comfortable, private space before they even attempt to touch the client. She also demonstrates how to enhance the possibility of experiencing pleasure. In short, you need to remove distractions and replace them with a wholehearted focus on feeling wonderful.

In any of the sensate focus exercises, or the moments alone when you explore sensual pleasure, conditioning makes it likely you will try to make something explosive happen for your partner or for yourself. That should come later. In the research phase, what you feel and how you feel it is the consuming emphasis of your activities. In your first moments as a sensual researcher, give yourself the opportunity to elicit some spine-tingling thrills through exploratory touching that has no endgame in mind.

If you follow the progression of sensate focus exercises, you might want to use the Whipple-Ogden matrix as a guide to the first series of exercises, which all involve non-genital touching. According to the Cornell University Health Services, begin by removing all clothing and jewelry, bathing, and then having one partner lie on his or her back with the other partner touching everything except the genitals, and varying the type of touch as suggested by Whipple and Ogden. In their 1994 book *Heterosexuality*, Masters, Johnson, and their colleague Robert C. Kolodny summarized the aim of the first part of sensate focus exercises as follows:

> The point of sensate focus is not to give your partner a back rub or massage (although either may be a perfectly wonderful and romantic thing to do on another occasion) or to touch her in a way that you think will make her happy. The point is very straightforward: to allow the person doing the touching to take in a variety of sensory experiences and to notice what they feel like, without any distractions or "should" lurking in the background.[4]

A complete description of the activities in non-genital touching is provided as a free download by Cornell Health Services.[5]

Step 3: Learn how to communicate what you've discovered.

Knowing what feels good, neutral, or awful is the easy part. For most people, describing that sensation is the hard part—but it is a key element of being in tune with pleasure. I briefly worked with a couple of top chefs on their book projects and was stunned at how my mouth watered just reading their menus. Their ability to convey flavor with words is a skill they learned as they were discovering how to combine flavors and master the art of cooking—just as you will learn how to convey feelings with works as you practice being a sensual researcher.

Elizabeth Gilbert, author of *Eat, Pray, Love*, is not a chef, but her experience of heavenly food lifted her ability to describe it in the book. In this paragraph, she describes the rapture of eating superior pizza dough:

> The dough, it takes me half my meal to figure out, tastes more like Indian *naan* than like any pizza dough I'd ever tried. It's soft and chewy and yielding, but incredibly thin. I always thought we had two choices in our lives when it came to pizza crust—thin and crispy, or thick and doughy. How was I to have known there could be a crust in this world that was thin and doughy? Holy of holies! Thin, doughy, strong, gummy, yummy, chewy, salty pizza paradise.[6]

In *Children of the Mind,* science fiction writer Orson Scott Card evokes a specific sensation that may cause you go back in time to when you last stood on a beach barefoot:

> She worked her toes into the sand, feeling the tiny delicious pain of the friction of tiny chips of silicon against the tender flesh between her toes. That's life. It hurts, it's dirty, and it feels very, very good.[7]

Not everyone has the descriptive powers to create vivid sense-oriented sentences, of course, but everyone can draw from experience to communicate about how a certain touch feels. For example, if your partner's hand is cold and he rubs lotion on your back, you might say, "It feels like you're sliding an ice cream cone down my spine."

Experiment with communicating to yourself first, and then to your partner, about the exact characteristics of a sensation. Start with the basics like hot, cold, scratchy, tickly, soft, sharp, and so on, and then build on the basics to get more specific. And keep in mind that you help yourself improve as a sensual communicator by adding details to stories about non-intimate experiences you've had. If you've just ridden the Fahrenheit roller coast at Hersheypark, Pennsylvania, try providing details of every heart-stopping moment of the 85-second ride, especially the 97-degree drop and corkscrew turns.

You can use what you learn about building pleasurable sensations in your body throughout your life. And the communication of what is pleasurable enables you to bring more of that enjoyment everywhere you go—not just during an intimate experience, but also when you're cooking a meal together, strolling in a park, or offering each other a friendly "good morning" on a sunny day. A healthy relationship can go to a whole new level when the "communication of pleasure" seasons everyday conversation.

As a rule, clear communication about anything you consider relevant or important enhances a relationship. And even though you wouldn't want to divulge all your private thoughts or secrets, letting a few leak out over the years could sustain his curiosity about you: "What will I learn about her *next* year?"

Just after writing this section on communication, I happened to see a featured article on msn.com called "Shhh . . . 9 Secrets Women Keep from Men." The author admitted that, after ten years of marriage, she keeps these secrets and asked her readers if they agree "that women should guard these nine secrets from their partners like the Secret Service guards a president."[8] It will come as no surprise that this is one reader who disagreed with her on most of them:

> We have facial hair.
> We pleasure ourselves, too.
> It wasn't great for us.
> We fart.
> How much we weigh.
> Our number of past partners.
> We're still hungry after that salad.
> That thing we asked you to do? We can do it ourselves.
> We need you.

Whether you're twenty-five or seventy-five, go ahead and admit the truth about most of these things to your partner. Chatting about at least three of them could lead to considerable pleasure. Blaming the dog for your bad odors is okay, though.

Step 4: Notice changes in your body and attitude as you experience different types of pleasure.

There are two ways to interpret this step. The first is paying attention to the subtle, or not-so-subtle, variances in the way your body responds to different pleasurable stimuli. The second involves broadening your definition of "pleasure"—calling experiences "pleasure" that you had considered either neutral or annoying—and then noticing your physical and emotional responses.

Yvonne Wray, an instructor with The Welcomed Consensus, expressed fear, apprehension, and denial when she first realized she was perimenopausal. That negative viewpoint started to change when she committed to experiencing menopause with as much pleasure as possible. Wray's professional background is computer science. She is a practical, logical person who recognizes that a pleasurable life supports health and happiness a great deal more than a life corroded by anxiety, complaints, and trauma. Her blog posts reflect her practical, logical nature; it's easy to track with her as she charts the mental and emotional shifts toward pleasure in her blog posts on menopause. One of the opening posts is "Help for Menopause: How I Got Relief and Gained Happiness," and it concludes with this:

I no longer felt like a victim of nature. I was making choices that directly and positively impacted my happiness. I was paying attention to my body in a new way, without the dread and fear. I was coming up, out of the dark and life was back in my hands. Going for the fun continues to be an invaluable tool that I use to guide my actions every day while going through the tremendous changes that accompany menopause.[9]

That was all well and good until Wray realized that hot flashes would likely be part of her experience of menopause for the foreseeable future. It was a rude awakening that there might be moments she would *not* call pleasurable, and certainly not call fun. She had to transform her mindset if she was going to realize her goal of a pleasurable menopause.

You must do something active and intentional in order to have something as disruptive as hot flashes become a path to pleasure. Once you make that decision, you can change the conversation in your head away from something that says, "Menopause symptoms are bad or something to avoid or tolerate," to "I can do things to capitalize on what is pleasurable about this experience."[10]

Wray had been in menopause for a number of years, with the hot flashes not abating, when she consulted her mother. She had not done any hormone therapy or taken any bioidenticals, so nature was simply moving her body along an unaltered track. Her mother had hot flashes for more than a decade—it's not uncommon that women experience them that long—so Wray decided she had to find a way to go past coping and actually enjoy them. This is a true Welcomed Consensus perspective on finding pleasure that a menopausal woman with disruptive symptoms might think is impossible to adopt. It is not impossible; what Wray did can be replicated.

Her thoughts in the blog post about the turnaround were inspiring, but the way she discovered how to enjoy hot flashes is not just revolutionary, it is also physiologically valid. Here are excerpts from her blog post called "Down for the Count" that track how she went from miserable to joyous in twenty seconds:

Time slows down. I realize what is coming and my brain races. *"Oh NOOOoooooo!"* that first reaction despondently echoes within me. I brace for what I know is next. The first rumblings make themselves known. I don't like this. I feel myself going down, slumber erased from

my world in a snap. I don't have much time. My heart is already racing.
. . .

I lay still. The silence outside my body remains unbroken, but inside
there is an outcry, *"Arrrrgggghhhhhh."* For whatever reason, that
thinking, judging part of me does not handle this recurring event very
well. . . .

I decide to feel my body, pay attention to it. I'm naked, lying on my
right side, hips and knees curled. My body is tense. One hand grips the
corner of my pillow. I relax, letting my fingers unfurl. . . . I relax even
more and *Lub-WHUMP* a single robust heartbeat reverberates loudly in
my chest. Seemingly in answer, a new thought pops into my consciousness. *"Count the seconds,"* and so I do.[11]

At this point in the blog post, Wray devotes two paragraphs to vividly
describing the heat building in her body and pushing outward to create
rivulets of sweat. In reading those paragraphs, it would be easy to get
the sense that she suffered excruciating heat for five or ten minutes. She
concludes the description with, "I am still counting. I've only reached
nine."[12] Nine seconds marks the turning point of her perception of what
a hot flash represents. She continues:

I am in awe at the capabilities of the human body, at my body! The movement and release of energy continues and I am like a kid looking forward
to what will happen next in a new action flick. . . .

The temperature peaks and I feel the beginning of its rapid fall. At
fifteen seconds there is so much perspiration happening all at once that
the surface of my skin feels dewy, **glowing as if I just stepped out of
a steamy shower**. Vapor rises, a layer of tropical atmosphere hovers
around me. The pressure from the inside subsides. I am aware of the
rhythm of my heart, slower with each beat. Inside my body the roar-
ing heat has dissipated. I breathe in deeply. . . . I feel the last remaining
threads of heat waft from the top of my head as I whisper the count to
myself—*"Twenty."* . . .

During those twenty seconds, I'd crossed the line. That hot flash *was
fun. Pleased, I turn over, fluff up my pillows*, and drift back to sleep.[13]

A couple of women commenting on the blog post felt motivated to
try Wray's approach and affirmed that it worked for them. It is likely,
however, that someone experiencing a ten-minute hot flash instead of a
twenty-second one would have a greater challenge sustaining a positive
attitude.

During our interview for this book, Wray added that some of the same sensations she had during the hot flash are sensations she has during peak sexual experiences. It is true that rushes of heat go through the body and that there is often visible flushing during orgasm—just as a woman would experience during a hot flash. In Wray's case, adopting a radically unusual viewpoint about a despised symptom of menopause helped her create an exciting and pleasurable "new normal."

Step 5: Be deliberate about your pleasure.

The concept of Deliberate Orgasm (DOing) is central to Welcomed Consensus teaching, which encourages women to establish "DO dates." As noted in the previous chapter, the clitoris has the highest concentration of nerve endings in the body—eight thousand, or roughly double that of the penis—and DOing emphasizes the pleasure possibilities of that fact by having the clitoris stroked directly. DO dates celebrate a connection with your partner and a connection with yourself that is 100 percent about the goal of pleasure. And since DO dates ideally include talking about specific sensations each of you experienced during the date, communication between you and your partner should take on a new dimension. It's time to put aside conversation about house repairs and investment returns and plunge into fun.

Your appreciation of the value of your own pleasure is the most vital viewpoint you can adopt to establish a "new normal" during and after menopause.

THE GATEWAYS TO A NEW VIEWPOINT

Having worked very closely with both psychotherapists and psychiatrists, I have come to the conclusion that there are two gateway feelings for a fabulous, fulfilling relationship with yourself and with your partner. These are essential elements in discovering or restoring true, vibrant intimacy: a sense of safety and the willingness to be vulnerable. Trevor Crow Mullineaux, with whom I wrote *Forging Healthy Connections* and *Blending Families*, particularly helped shape my convictions about these gateway perceptions. Together, we explored research underlying much of her clinical approach to family and couples' counseling, which is rooted in emotionally focused therapy. Emotionally focused therapy is considered a short-term therapy, effective in helping couples take steps toward creating a secure bond.

A SENSE OF SAFETY

Feeling safe is a critical part of turning the menopause and postmenopause years into enjoyable ones. A sense of security is not a state to be avoided, despite what pop culture might have us believe. Rather, it's a healthful way to live and the natural and desired outcome of strong connections with other human beings. The positive, physical effects of a secure relationship do powerful and practical things for our bodies and our sense of risk-taking and competence. They prepare us to have more pleasure enter our lives.

Consider the internal physiological effect of not feeling safe. In a sado-masochistic experience, feeling unsafe is erotic—but most of us do not want a high-risk sexual experience involving pain. Threat of physical harm is not a source of pleasure; it is a source of abject fear. The symptoms of that fear churn within us and slam shut pleasure responses that have been described earlier in this chapter. A major fear response is that blood flows to the reptilian (survival) and mammalian (emotion) brain at the expense of the primate (cognitive) brain. You obviously cannot communicate what feels good to you in an intimate encounter—a DO date—if your cognitive abilities are impaired.

A fear response actually makes you sick, so if your partner suggests that going toward a pain experience is erotic, tell him/her two things: (1) *Fifty Shades of Grey* is a really bad book, and (2) no.

On the flip side, a belief that your partner is a source of safety and security has a profoundly positive effect on physiological responses. University of Virginia psychologist Dr. James Coan's 2006 study published in the *Journal of Psychological Science* illustrates the effect of a positive connection with another human being on the fear response.[14] Using functional magnetic resonance imaging to track their brain activity, Coan administered small electric shocks to sixteen married women whenever they saw an "X" flash before them. The women's brains lit up when they felt the shock and were alone. The response diminished when a stranger held their hand. It plummeted when holding the hand of their husband. The women in the happiest relationships felt the most relief.

Regardless of how you define or practice a "happy relationship," you are better off in terms of the quality of your intimate interaction if you feel safe and so does your partner. A mutually protective relationship gives you the benefit of ideal physiological responses to a range of pleasures. The physical and mental health benefits of feeling safe are enormous and well-documented, warding off attacks on the immune system and cognitive abilities so you are better prepared to enjoy health, connection, and communication with your partner.

COMMITMENT TO VULNERABILITY

Vulnerability is a vital ingredient to connecting intimately with another human being. It is vital in enduring love. In fact, if we turn to insights from the author most known for her serious research into vulnerability, professor Brené Brown (*Daring Greatly*), we could easily shape an argument that vulnerability is essential in enabling a woman to create a pleasurable menopause and postmenopause.

In 2010, Brown gave a TEDx Talk in Houston called "The Power of Vulnerability" that was so popular, it scored millions of views over the next few weeks. Offers to speak poured in from sources as diverse as parent-teacher groups to Fortune 500 companies. Ironically, many of those company executives that called her complimented her talk out of one side of their mouth and asked her *not* to talk about vulnerability out of the other. She asked them what she should talk about if not her area of expertise. Their response: innovation, creativity, and change.

In a 2012 follow-up mainstage TED Talk, Brown told the audience what she told the executives: "Vulnerability is the birthplace of innovation, creativity, and change. To create is to make something that has never existed before. There's nothing more vulnerable than that. Adaptability to change is all about vulnerability."[15] Sounds like a game plan for a woman intent on moving well through major life changes.

As part of your shift in viewpoint that helps you shape a "new normal," it would be useful to reverse your negative thinking about what vulnerability means. A lot of people see it like an open window that lets germs and fumes into your lungs. Instead, think of it as an open window that allows fresh air to fill your lungs and cool breezes to invigorate you.

Vulnerability and a sense of safe haven go hand in hand in relationships. The way you know that you can begin to enjoy vulnerability with another person is by paying attention to signals from your body. The autonomic nervous system detects threats as well as the absence of threats. Start by determining if you have any anxiety when you're with your partner in an intimate situation. If so, where in your body do you feel it?

Millie was a gymnast in high school, and her coach gave her an insight that ultimately affected her life. Her coach observed that Millie would put tension into her shoulders whenever she was attempting a new move or felt challenged with a routine she was doing. Time after time, she heard, "Drop your shoulders!" The muscles in and around her shoulders were where she stored performance anxiety.

Many years later, Millie thought about this when she realized her shoulders were tense when she was in an intimate situation with her husband. She wasn't physically or emotionally afraid of him or concerned about being judged by him. The raised shoulders and muscle spasm exhibited the performance burden she was putting on herself. She communicated what she noticed to him, and just doing that drained the tension from her shoulders. Millie could start forming a new point of view that integrated a feeling of safety and enjoyment of vulnerability.

Pay attention to your body, and what triggers feelings of pleasure or discomfort, as you try to shape your viewpoint about a "new normal" in your intimate life. Let your mind wander: If you have menopause symptoms pretty much under control—or are well past them—what adventures lie ahead? And what can you do to make them happen?

Exercise: What do you need? What do you want?

In his bestselling book, *The Five Love Languages*, Gary Chapman poses simple questions and thoughts to the reader within each chapter devoted to one of the five "languages." The love languages he delves into are words of affirmation, quality time, receiving gifts, acts of service, and physical touch. Inspired by these five love languages as described by Chapman,[16] I have created a playful exercise designed to remind you of what you need and want from your partner to help boost desire, a sense of intimacy, and ultimately the enjoyment of pleasure—*your* pleasure:

- What would you most like to hear your partner say to you when you are making love?
- What invitation would you most like to hear from your partner to create quality time together?
- Even if finances are tight, what gift would you most like to receive from your partner?
- Many acts of service involve household chores, but not all. What are some non-chore ways your partner might "serve" you that would delight you?
- Recall some nonsexual "touching times" that enhanced intimacy between the two of you. What made these times special? What do you want to do again?

Chapter Eight

Applying the Knowledge

Patti and Bob married when he was eighty-two and she was seventy-eight. They had known each for more than fifty years and had both lost their spouses a few years before. Pat was very slim and fit and had a prescription for Premarin cream that helped her get ready for her wedding night. Yes, they consummated their relationship, and did not mind strongly hinting about it the next day when they were having brunch with family and friends. Raised eyebrows and muffled giggles suggested that at least a few of the people at the party didn't think that such "elderly" people were capable of sex.

In a 2018 study, the American Association of Retired Persons (AARP) concluded that Patti and Bob are not that unusual, particularly because their intimate relationship was relatively new. The survey AARP conducted in conjunction with the University of Michigan involved 1,002 people aged sixty-five to eighty years, and it revealed that 40 percent of them were still sexually active. The online survey I conducted as part of the research for this book covered women only from forty-five to eighty years, and exactly 50 percent of the respondents indicated that "sexual activity of any kind" was either "extremely important" or "very important" to their relationship. Supporting that inclination, 57 percent ranked their partner very high in terms of sexual appeal to them.

My survey did not specifically address the question of how interested the women were in sex—and that's a somewhat different issue from how important it is in the relationship. The AARP survey did address that question, however.

While the overall survey results from the AARP effort were broad-cast as good news for the mature population, their findings on interest in sex stood out for me as less than thrilling. Even though the percentage of people in the age group who were having sex was unexpectedly high, there was a significant gender imbalance in terms of *interest* in sex. Whereas half of the sixty-five- to eighty-year-old men who participated in the survey said they were "extremely or very interested in sex,"[1] only 12 percent of the women in that age group said they were interested.

Alison Bryant, senior vice president of research for AARP declared, "This survey just confirms that the need for and interest in sexual intimacy doesn't stop at a certain age."[2] That would seem to be true for men, but extrapolating from the data presented, one might conclude that many women with no interest in sex are having it anyway—presumably because their partner is in the 50 percent of men who are interested.

On a physiological level, that can be healthy. However, on a psychological and emotional level, it may not be.

The postmenopausal phase is where so many women give up sexuality and only want "closeness." That's fine. Intimacy can definitely be enjoyed without sex. The problem is that, without intercourse or sex acts that simulate intercourse, the vagina will not get the exercise it needs to stay healthy. As Dr. Hope Ricciotti, a gynecologist who teaches at Harvard Medical School says, "The vagina is a 'use it or lose it' place. The act of having intercourse stimulates blood flow to the vagina and keeps it healthy."[3]

With that in mind, we can say that the practical value of intercourse after menopause is certainly clear, and of course, we already know the mechanics. But why do it from a psychological and emotional perspective? That is the question that 88 percent of the women in the survey obviously don't have a good answer for.

The techniques of enjoyment in this chapter are paths to answering the question "Why do it?" They address the desire for and pleasurable experience of erotic love.

In her inspiring and energizing video course "Rekindling Desire," Esther Perel makes many provocative statements about why we lose desire for sex. She notes, "Part of why people lose their interest in sex is because they actually lose the erotic dimension of the sex."[4] They have either fallen into, or consciously opted for, a cozy relationship and collapsed the eroticism in the relationship—the mystery, the surprise, the adventure—down to nothing. In essence, they have lost their curiosity about what is possible with the other person they know so well. Even worse, they have lost their curiosity about the person. No matter how well couples think they know each other, there can still be surprises.

For five years, I worked on a book called *Government of All the People* with Robert L. Saloschin, who was known in the Department of Justice as the "Wizard of FOIA" (Freedom of Information Act). He was a brilliant constitutional lawyer who spent most of his career at the Department of Justice and rose to a senior level in the department. I also considered him my "other father," since I had lived with the Saloschin family when I was in my early twenties. I would sit in the living room with him and my "other mother," his wife Neita. Toward the end of the book development process, I asked Bob if he had any more colorful stories about his Navy service during World War II. He told me about an evening on the base when the mood lightened significantly; a group of nurses had been given temporary quarters and they had a little social time with the sailors before they were flown out. Neita laughed and raised her eyebrows: "I've never heard *that* story before!" At that point, they had already been married sixty-three years!

In short, never assume you know all of your spouse's stories, aspirations, opinions, and items on their bucket list no matter how many years you've been together. Take Perel's advice and remain curious as a way of staying connected to the adventure in your relationship.

The following sets of suggestions, weaving in tried-and-true advice from relationship experts and therapists, are designed to help you get in the mood for an intimate encounter, as well as to explore and enjoy the erotic dimension of intimacy.

Start by diminishing the anxiety, frustrations, or nagging doubts you may have that would get in the way of intimacy. And be honest with yourself about the anxiety you might have about engaging in an intimate encounter with your loved one—no matter how long you've been together. You also want to launch this new phase of your intimate life by getting in touch with the behaviors and body language that signal your true emotional state.

TAKE THE ELEVATOR

In his book *Arousal: The Secret Logic of Sexual Fantasies*, clinical psychologist Michael J. Bader notes that certain mood states are incompatible with arousal. When you are in a state of high stress, or experiencing a sense of fear or anger, then you cannot experience pleasure. A pervasive sense of anxiety does not allow you feel playful in a way that allows for enjoyable intimacy.

Trevor Crow Mullineaux, who is a relationship expert and my co-author on two books, uses something emotionally focused therapists call "bringing the elevator down." This is a couples' exercise used to de-escalate tension, but you could use a version of it as you mentally prepare yourself to engage in an intimate encounter. The idea is to put yourself in a calm state, leaving behind the tensions, annoyances, and even anger that may have built up during the day.

In a session with a couple, the action would be having one member of the couple air the reasons why he or she feels angry, frustrated, or hurt, with the other person genuinely engaging through non-judgmental listening. In this case, you would listen to yourself—really listen to yourself. I found myself in a state of very high stress recently and tried this: I sat in a tub of hot water and listened to myself silently explain why I was feeling that way. I could feel the elevator come down to the ground floor.

Once at the ground floor, you can start taking the elevator back up—but this time, to a high-energy, feel-good state. One technique is to consider all you have to be grateful for.

In his book, *The Mood Elevator*, Dr. Larry Senn puts gratitude at the top of the mood elevator.

> There are a few reasons, but the first one is that gratitude is an overriding emotion. It is almost impossible to be both grateful and depressed at the same time. There is a sense of calm, warmth, and happiness that comes with gratitude that overrides impatience, frustration, and anger. Gratitude is also a perspective and a decision—a decision to practice looking at what we do appreciate about our lives and other people versus looking at what we lack.[5]

Where to start? Right now, you could send your loving partner a text saying, "I just had an important thought: You're wonderful and I appreciate you!"

LOCATE YOUR FEELINGS

The following insight and exercise on "felt sense" also comes from Trevor Mullineaux and the realm of emotionally focused therapy. They center on identifying where you feel certain emotions so that you are more self-aware about your expressions of them as well as better able to signal your partner about how you express them. It builds on the story of Millie, the gymnast in chapter 7 who stored tension in her shoulders.

When Mullineaux asks clients to locate a certain feeling in their bodies, they typically look at her with skepticism. Their first reaction is usually "Are you serious?" Some say, "In my heart," if the feeling is lost love. For most feelings, however, the idea of making a visceral connection to an emotion is completely foreign to many people.

Most of us don't acknowledge or honor that all our emotions are first felt physically. When we are afraid, we feel it by our hearts beating faster and our breaths getting shallower. All emotions—sadness, happiness, shame, disgust—are first registered in our bodies. As an emotionally focused therapist, Mullineaux's job is often to guide clients through the "felt sense" of events.

If a physician asked you, "Where does it hurt?" or "Where does it itch?" you could probably give an answer without hesitation. In putting the concept of "felt sense" to work in your life, you will be making the same kind of link between emotion and your body—and you will give yourself and your loved one(s) a powerful tool to support health and healing.

For example, Mullineaux might ask a husband, "When your wife tells you she appreciates what you do for her, where do you feel it?" He might respond, "I feel it in my shoulders, maybe more relaxed." He describes how he feels more at ease or safer within the relationship at that moment. That is his felt sense of her regard for him. Let's say that recognition of felt sense started happening on a regular basis—for both of them. He's tremendously stressed out from something that happens at the office. She sees that his shoulders are raised and maybe his arms are drawn in tightly to his body. She tells him how grateful she and the kids are for what he does, especially knowing what he has to put up with sometimes. Shoulders down, he immediately starts to de-stress.

In the context of an intimate relationship, love as a felt sense involves the other person's body and mind as much as it involves yours. A loving couple doesn't feel love *for* each other; they feel love *in* each other. Love, therefore, is the felt sense that you exist in the heart, mind, and soul of another person. It is not a lofty concept but a humble one. It is also essentially an erotic one, capturing the image of being pleasurable inside one another.

Consider how the concept of synchronicity is central to understanding/feeling this definition of love. This is about a patterned, rhythmic connection with another person—someone with whom we have laid down positive neurological pathways in our brain.

The difficulty some people have in grasping this definition is that sources typically define it intellectually as an outgoing emotion—one that a person experiences and projects. According to the Merriam-Webster dictionary, love is:

1. strong affection for another arising out of kinship or personal ties [maternal love for a child]
2. attraction based on sexual desire: affection and tenderness felt by lovers
3. affection based on admiration, benevolence, or common interests [love for his old schoolmates].[6]

In contrast to those "push" definitions of love, the definition we'll use here focuses on the incoming nature of love. It is the experience of your existence in another person's mind and heart.

To get a personal sense of what "felt sense" means in your relationship, try this exercise:

- Think of the last time your partner/spouse did something kind and caring for you. Feel where it rests in your body as you recall it.
  - Does your heart feel bigger?
  - Can you breathe deeper?
  - Is there less stress in your shoulders?
  - Anything else?

Try to feel a positive experience in your body and think about that for a few moments. Expand on it. When we have the "felt sense" that we are safe, that we are loved, valued, and known, we have less tension in our bodies. We can actually feel the experience in our physical beings.

- Now think of a time that you were under attack. Maybe your partner criticized you for doing something hurtful or selfish. Where did you experience that in your body? Try to locate the physicality of the moment.
  - Did your stomach churn?
  - Did you feel like your breathing was restricted?
  - Did you tense up your shoulders or your fists?
  - Anything else?

Making contact with the bodily experience of emotion is vitally important to understanding your emotions. The more aware of your own physical process you can become, the more you can share it with your partner. The more your partner grasps the connection for you, the better he or she is able to help you thrive.

STICK WITH THE "WORKOUT"

In 1997 and 1998, I had the opportunity to collaborate on an exercise and nutrition book with an amazing fitness expert named Patrick "Sarge" Avon. I had been a competitive athlete in a number of sports, so I knew the language and principles of fitness. But I had no credentials other than a few trophies. So I studied diligently and took one of the hardest tests of my adult life, the American Council on Exercise test, to become a certified personal trainer. In 1998, I earned that designation and have maintained it; it's a source of immense pride for me. Every two years, I need to take a series of courses and tests to stay current with my knowledge and have found myself gravitating toward the courses that plunge me into the techniques of motivation. I apply them to myself when I don't feel like going to gym—and they work.

In my opinion, the same techniques that get a lazy body to the gym, or just outside for a walk around the block, are those that anyone can use to increase the commitment to rekindled desire and intimacy. They are also techniques that emphasize the enjoyment of the activity. I have never embraced the mantra "No pain, no gain." My training has always been, "No pain, more fun."

SCHEDULE TIME

One of the worst pieces of relationship advice I've ever heard came from the sister of a friend of mine. My friend felt her husband was "bugging her" about having more sex. Her sister said, "Just say, 'yes.' Heck, what's five minutes out of your life once or twice a week?"

Taking that advice means you turn a sexual encounter into a job. It's like the five minutes you take to clean the stovetop or start a load of laundry. Would any woman really look forward to sex as a household chore?

When we were twenty-five years old and dating, spontaneous hooking up was a thrilling prospect. Even at fifty-five, it might be a thrilling prospect if you're a widow or divorcee. But for most of us, spontaneity and sex do not go well together. We have been with the same person for a few decades and, frankly, the thrill isn't the same hot fire it used to be. So, to raise the heat, we need to schedule time for erotic love—a time to relax and play together—and never treat it like a routine household chore.

If that sounds boring, then consider all of the fun things you do in a month that are on your calendar, whether that schedule is stored in your head or captured on your smartphone. You get together with two other couples once a month for cocktails. You don't know if it will be a Wednesday or a Thursday or whether it will be 5:00 or 5:30, but you know it will happen. Your women's group meets once a month to plan your charity work and, depending on the time of day, it might be a coffee date or a happy hour. You and your spouse watch a half-hour sitcom every Thursday night at 8. And then there's one of your favorite things: Sunday morning, you go to the local recreation center for your long cardio workout. Almost no one else is there. You have your choice of treadmill, rowing machine, or bike. You can have any lane in the lap pool. There's no one there to watch you hit balls badly at the golf simulator. It's like the taxpayers of your town built this rec center just for you!

Obviously, scheduling fun events can get your juices flowing, so why would scheduling time for intimacy be any different? If anything, it makes it special.

The Welcomed Consensus, introduced in the last chapter, encourages couples to set up DO dates, that is, Deliberate Orgasm dates. These are times in which the couple focuses on peak intimate experiences. The aim is fun. Pleasure, pure pleasure! For a kid, the equivalent would be going to the community pool with friends—we could hardly wait until Memorial Day when we could go every day the sun poked through.

Scheduling does not need to entail putting intimacy on your calendar from 3:15 to 4:00, the way you would log a doctor's appointment or conference call, of course. It might be more a matter of knowing that you both have flexible schedules on the weekends, so Sunday afternoon tends to be a relaxed few hours where you can mentally slot in time for play. That kind of scheduling is more in keeping with how Perel says that erotic couples behave: They have "routines and signs of avail-ability"[7] that are part of what help them sustain and fuel their intimacy.

TAKE OWNERSHIP

If you give in to the thinking, "It's just five minutes out of your week!" then you give your partner total control over your sex life. You abdicate any responsibility for pleasure and admit overtly that having sex is not about you. All you do is show up.

Part of taking ownership is the planning and preparation you invest in intimate times with your partner. You prepare for the cocktail party with your friends by assembling a plate of appetizers. You prepare for watching the Thursday night sitcom with your husband by making a bowl of popcorn. When it comes time for your rendezvous with your loved one, you might want to grab the lube and spend a few moments warming up your engine so you're in the mood for fun. Pairing that with reading a few pages of Mary Roach's *Bonk* may get you aroused and make you laugh at the same time.

A companion part of ownership involves communication: being explicit about what you find pleasurable and what you don't. If you had a personal trainer at your gym and he kept dictating how you did your workout, you would probably speak up. And if he didn't listen to you, you might stop showing up. The first time you try communicat-ing about sex with your partner, it may be difficult—or even close to impossible—to express yourself clearly. In all likelihood, however, it will get easier. The alternative is that you will not be inclined to show for your date.

That brings us to the next element of developing a great "workout"—being patient with yourself when it comes to erotic love goals.

GIVE YOURSELF TIME TO
ACHIEVE YOUR GOALS

The overarching goal is probably mutual pleasure—so sublime it could make the sun come out at night. Right? Well, at the very least the goal is mutual pleasure that gives you a definite sense that your relationship is still alive and well. Depending on how long it's been since you had regular intimate relations, this might take time. Even if you've been having maintenance sex—which is not an inherently bad thing—you might need lots of transition time to move your intimacy to new heights and forms of pleasure.

You would never expect yourself to lose ten pounds the first time you work out. Don't make equally unreasonable demands on your first few weeks of trying to reconnect physically and sensually with your partner. As menopausal or postmenopausal women, probably with partners who have as many sags and wrinkles as we do, just getting used to using our bodies in an erotic way again can be challenging on many levels.

At the same time, it's always good to remind yourself that you're moving forward. One thing that has worked well for Jim and me is to do a playful "debrief." It's not a matter of comparing one date to another, but rather pointing out something special, funny, or interesting that we think is worth calling out.

It also never hurts to give a genuine compliment and express appreciation that your partner set aside time to focus on your relationship. It means you've met the most important goal of all: spending pleasurable time together.

MAKE IT PERSONAL

This is about your pleasure and shared erotic love. It is not about how sexy you look, or don't look, in a pink negligee. It's also not about how many times your partner yells, "Oh, God!"

Consider all the sensual elements that might enhance the experience for you: the temperature of the room, music, the fact that it's day rather than night (or vice versa), the brand of lube you choose, whether it's important to have freshly washed hair, turning the phones off, and so on. Keep a record of what worked for you and what didn't so that you can repeat the good and eliminate the rest.

Making it personal respects your lover as well. You bring more of yourself to the experience when you have the elements in place that excite both of you. Not to stereotype, but women do have a tendency to be other-focused and too much of that can undermine your ability to fully experience your own pleasure. Blogger and author Winona

Dimeo-Ediger calls this "happiness by proxy,"[8] and it is best left behind during intimate times with your lover—who will likely have more fun knowing that you feel satisfied.

TAKE PRIDE

In the movies, it often seems as though the sex is so hot and the stars are so gorgeous that the rest of us must stink at lovemaking and not be worth looking at naked. We need to remember that Sharon Stone and Michael Douglas had the benefit of director Paul Verhoeven to help choreograph their passion in *Basic Instinct.*

People have a natural aversion to doing things they think they do badly, especially if they think they do them badly all the time. In golf, one good shot in a round keeps people coming back. But if there's not even one good shot, the clubs will go to Goodwill unless the golfer focuses on the sunshine, soft grass, and relaxing walk.

Smile and confidently move toward pleasure. Don't try to be Brad Pitt and Angelina Jolie in *Mr. and Mrs. Smith.* We all know that didn't turn out so well in the long run anyway.

SAMPLE THE CHEESECAKE

Sex therapist Dr. Jenni Skyler contributes some wonderful insights into the thriving sexual lives of clients from a young age to nearly ninety. She originated the term *Cheesecake of Pleasure* to describe the many sexually fulfilling options that a couple might explore in addition to, or instead of, intercourse.

She hotly criticizes the medical characterization of the sexual response cycle that breaks the experience into four phases: excitement, plateau, orgasm, and resolution. Instead, she is much more in tune with others cited in this book who looked at full-bodied enjoyment of sensuality, the possibility of sustained orgasm, and movement in and out of phases.

> We want to redefine sex as a more holistic and comprehensive under-standing of sensual contact. When we change our minds about the defini-tion of sex, we change how we behave as intimate beings with each other.[9]

The standard performance-oriented concept in a sexual encounter is profoundly male-oriented: kiss, take your clothes off, have genital contact, have intercourse, have an orgasm, relax. That might work for young women—although it's arguable how well it works for most young women—but it's a terrible progression for a mature woman because it does not reflect the model of how women achieve the greatest satisfaction in a sexual encounter. It is a medical process, not the experience of erotic love.

Offered freely online from The Welcomed Consensus, the "30 Day Pleasure Challenge"[10] is a tool to get you ready to experiment with Skyler's Cheesecake of Pleasure. It involves building from one minute of sensual pleasure up to thirty minutes over the course of a month. The experience is meant for you—to stimulate your senses and your sense awareness—even if you have a partner.

Pick one or more categories of sense experience and focus on it for an incremental number of minutes—one to thirty—taking a rest day every ten days:

- Sight: Look outside at trees blowing in the breeze, a favorite piece of art, cloud formations
- Smell: Take in the aroma of freshly baked cookies, the sweet smell of flowers
- Taste: Savor a cup of peppermint tea, a piece of chocolate, buttery brie on a cracker
- Sound: Listen to a favorite song, birds singing to you, the purr of your cat
- Touch: Enjoy the warmth of your shower water, the soft feel of your bathrobe, lotion on your feet
- Conceptual thought: Read a couple of pages of an erotic novel, watch the Welcomed Consensus video on "The Three-Minute Orgasm" online

After each session, make a note or two about the sensation that day. At the end of the thirty days, stage a celebration that lasts thirty minutes—whatever tickles your senses.

Consistent with the focus on pleasure rather than orgasm, the Cheesecake of Pleasure is an intimacy model that we might call a "tasting experience," with each activity delivering an enjoyable sensation. These are the possible elements of the model that Saketh Guntupalli and I developed with Skyler for the book *Sex and Cancer*:

1. Prepare to share the cheesecake by having a solo date. Know your own body so you know what you're sharing with your partner.
2. Know what turns you on mentally. Get to know the literature and film that ignites your sexual fantasies.
3. Engage in sensual massage.
4. Engage in sensual massage involving the genitals.
5. Have a kissing date. Everything you do is kissing from head to toe.
6. Caress the genitals with your hands.
7. Caress the genitals with your mouth.
8. Cook together. Enjoying the many textures and flavors of food can be erotic.
9. Play with the genitals. A little vibration, a smooth move . . .
10. Indulge in intercourse using a lot of lube.
11. Indulge in intercourse with various positions.
12. Find exotic places to have sex, whether or not it's intercourse, like the car or in the bedroom at your sister's house.
13. Have fun with lube. There are so many different kinds, and each can promote pleasure in a unique way.
14. Have fun with toys.[11]

Skyler guides her clients through the tasting experience by suggesting that each "slice of cheesecake" might get at least fifteen minutes, with the only ground rule being that both members of the couple agree to each one.

> My only rule is enthusiastic consent. Example flavors can be sensual massage, sensual showers, mutual masturbation, intercourse, manual stimulation, oral sex, anal sex, play with dildos, play with vibrators, play with blindfolds, and on and on.[12]

As with all of the other activities in this book, your body is central to the experience, and is the vehicle for pleasure, but the pleasure springs from your mind.

Chapter Nine

The Force of Lifestyle Changes

In the movie *Thor: Ragnarok*, Thor, son of Odin, who is the size of a normal man, goes up against the Incredible Hulk. The match is a little like a woman doing battle against Time. Thor is a god, of course, so he has special powers, just as we goddesses do. Even so, Hulk is so, well, incredible, that even banging into him full force will only make you exhausted. You will never win. The equal and opposite reaction is that you are pushed back as hard as you pushed. Darned third law of Newton!

Menopause is a time for finesse, for lifestyle changes that acknowledge the unstoppable force of time and slow it down, not fight it. It is a time to channel your strength to achieve satisfaction of all kinds instead of putting energy into going head-to-head with the Hulk known as Time.

Previous chapters featured myriad pieces of guidance on products, medicines, and actions that could help address symptoms of menopause and enhance your enjoyment of intimacy. This chapter spotlights essential lifestyle modifications, some of which were referenced before, but were not the point of focus. Menopause really is the "change of life," with some of our habits and preferences no longer appropriate in terms of health, appearance, and sexuality. The bitter reality is that some of the things that worked for us before in those areas no longer do, and some of them damage our health, appearance, and sexuality.

THE FORCE OF NUTRITION

In the early days of this century, I wrote a book about nutrition for competitive athletes. Realizing that it contained fundamentals of healthy eating, I reviewed the table of contents and saw that the key topics in the book are exactly the same topics that should be covered in a book on nutrition for women who are menopausal or postmenopausal. The difference is that the insights aren't helping you fuel a marathon run or lift a record amount of weight: they are helping you enhance the quality of a life as you deal with a body that is going through substantial changes.

Just like a competitive athlete, you need to know how to eat for energy, aid recovery, supplement for strength, add endurance, gain or cut weight, handle stressful conditions, and make sure your food is age-appropriate. And just like a competitive athlete, you need to do what the US Department of Agriculture finally did: scrap the food pyramid. That horrible illustration of "good" eating morphed a bit through the years, going from bad to less bad, but it never gave reasonable guidance on healthy eating. With the foundation layers of the pyramid being two forms of carbohydrates topped by dairy products, the food pyramid was a guide to gaining weight for menopausal women (and most other people as well).

Former First Lady Michelle Obama seemed happy to kick the food pyramid into history's trash bin and replace it with MyPlate, which does not emphasize a gluttonous amount of grain and dairy. Instead, the image is a plate split into four sections—a simple reminder that a balanced diet, with a little dairy on the side, is a reasonable approach. As nutritional science progresses, we may find that the portions are a bit off, but it's a major improvement over the notorious pyramid.

You may not agree with the scientific opinion of metabolic researcher Dr. Scott Connelly; however, I think it has great value as a thought-provoking launch point for a discussion of nutritional changes that have the power to improve your health and energy:

> There is no magical disconnect between evolution and metabolism. Our brain size and complexity reflect billions of years of evolution, but the liver is the same liver as 10,000 years ago when agriculture came into being. It's impossible to suggest that any significant genetic change has occurred at the level of metabolism to account and deal with the perversion of the natural food supply that has occurred, first and foremost with

agriculture. On top of that, 200 years ago industrialization brought processing into the picture. All of this has added up to task the system beyond its limits for metabolic transformation.

From the standpoint of what your system understands, the food pyramid is nonsense. Among the six food groups, two didn't exist throughout most of human history. Dairy and bread/cereals are not required.[1]

Quoting Connelly should not be construed as an endorsement of one of the trending diets that cuts out all dairy and grains. It's included as a reminder that heavy reliance on them is unwise from a metabolic standpoint. As much fun as it might be to live on cheese and crackers, with a glass of wine on the side, it would probably make your menopause nightmarish and boost your dress size. Increasing the intake of certain types of foods and decreasing others can affect the severity of menopause symptoms, hormone production, and your ability to make the most of actions you are taking to sustain your intimate life. In terms of weight, steady blood sugar levels, and quality sleep, it would be difficult to argue with the logic of eliminating or at least cutting down on doughnuts, bagels, sodas, and those fabulous Thin Mint Girl Scout cookies.

PRINCIPLES OF ENERGY

When you combine what you eat with oxygen, the output is carbon dioxide, water, and a chemical called adenosine triphosphate (ATP). ATP is the body's direct energy supply, a chemical substance required for all muscular activity, including sex.

Your body uses energy continuously, whether you are babysitting your infant granddaughter or sleeping. There is no "off" switch that tells your body processes to shut down and wait until the next meal. Among other requirements, your body continuously needs blood sugar to run the brain, the heart, and the kidneys. If you do not provide the raw materials that your biochemical factories require, your body will draw from other sources within it. The tissue most affected by this process is muscle.

Your muscle tissue already has huge responsibilities for keeping the body healthy—this is the only source of stored nitrogen, which is vital for basic functions like cell division—so asking it to make up for deficits in eating means loss of functionality. A basic concept in eating for energy, therefore, is that food you eat must serve your entire body's need for fuel, down to the cellular level. It is more than slurping a caffeine beverage and stomping off to your next commitment.

Carbohydrates, proteins, and fats all have a role in energy production. Carbs lead the way, though, as a ready source of fuel for both the body and the brain. Carbs are carbon and water (hydrogen and oxygen); fats are also carbon, hydrogen, and oxygen. Proteins consist of amino acids, also composed of carbon, oxygen, and hydrogen as well as nitrogen. In some cases, amino acids also contain sulfur. These latter elements set protein apart from the other nutrients in the role it plays in body functions.

Without carbohydrates in your system, your body will turn to the other two nutrients as fuel sources. Those other nutrients have jobs to do as well, and it is not a good idea to ask them to step away from those jobs to meet your energy needs. In brief, proteins have life-supporting functions, like fighting diseases, because antibodies and other elements support by the immune system are proteins. And you need fats to metabolize the fat-soluble vitamins A, D, E, and K. Just make sure your diet has all three nutrients. Specific guidelines on protein needs follow in the next section, so you might start by determining yours and build the rest of your diet around that calculation.

PROTEIN: ENERGY, RECOVERY, REPAIR

Protein needs increase with the onset of menopause. Because the body does not store protein—the way we know it stores fat—you need to increase your protein intake during menopause.

Protein is essential in terms of cell generation as well as cellular repair, so with the myriad changes going on in the body during menopause, getting sufficient protein is a significant wellness goal. Protein is a vital part of hormone and neurotransmitter synthesis; again, with all the changes inherent in menopause, skimping on protein can deprive of you of these substances you need for health and a positive state of mind. The short list of functions requiring protein that you become keenly aware of in menopause (and after) include hair and skin resilience, bone strength, your ability to make hormones of any kind, production of enzymes necessary for digestion, and generation of red blood cells to deliver iron and oxygen throughout the body. One of the women I interviewed who had some of the most unpleasant symptoms of menopause was a vegan. This is not to say that vegans are necessarily protein deprived, but vegans have to be more diligent than women with other dietary regimens to get a sufficient amount of protein to stay healthy during these changes.

Six of the red alerts for protein deficiency are:

- Edema. Swollen and puffy skin is not a symptom you are likely to see because this symptom indicates a severe deficiency. Unless you're living on cranberry juice and iceberg lettuce, you probably will not have edema from protein deficiency. You could have it, however, as a result of certain medications, a heart condition, kidney disease, or cirrhosis of the liver.
- Skin, hair, and nail problems. Hair thinning or hair loss are symptoms of menopause, but they are also symptoms of protein deficiency. Brittle nails and flaky skin can also signal it. Without getting sufficient protein, you will be exacerbating symptoms to which you are already predisposed.
- Weakness due to loss of muscle mass. In shortchanging yourself on dietary protein, tissues and organs related to critical body functions will "steal" it from your muscles. Keep in mind that a critical part of sexual health, not to mention continence, involves the muscles of the pelvic floor. When you think of "muscle mass," it would be a mistake to focus solely on thigh muscles and those triceps that can keep your arms from flapping like a flag in the breeze. Remember the muscles inside you that contribute to your quality of life (QOL).
- Weakened bones. You run a much greater risk of fractures with insufficient protein. Again, a woman who is menopausal or postmenopausal already runs the risk of osteoporosis, and starving your bones of protein will just ensure that you bring on bone trouble.
- Weakened immune system. Infections will be harder to fight off. One study focused specifically on older women who were kept on a low-protein diet for nine weeks; it documented "significant losses in lean tissue, immune response, and muscle function."[2]
- Insatiable hunger leading to weight gain. Mild protein deficiency prompts your body to crave more food. The easiest way to get a

sufficient number of protein calories is by eating animal protein. A menopausal woman who is a vegetarian or vegan is therefore likely to be the most susceptible to the trap of responding to the hunger with carbohydrates. Even too many healthy carbs will ensure weight gain.

Basic guidance on getting enough protein is that you should have it at every meal. How much you need on a daily basis depends both on your body weight and your level and type of activity. The general guideline is that you need 0.4 grams of protein for each pound of body weight; however, the need increases slightly as you age. A premenopausal woman weighing 135 pounds needs roughly fifty-four grams of protein; a 165-pound woman needs roughly sixty-six grams of protein. Around age fifty, you want to increase the amount to about 0.5 grams of protein per pound.

Here is where we can start to see the traps and nonsense of the now-defunct food pyramid. Let's say you are a fifty-five-year-old woman who has had a hearty, heart-healthy breakfast of oatmeal and you threw some blueberries on top as well as a little milk. That's seven grams of protein between the oatmeal and the milk, with the milk contributing some saturated fat. You have a turkey breast (five ounces) sandwich on whole grain bread for lunch—mustard, some lettuce and tomato. That's about twenty-eight grams of protein, and you congratulate yourself on having no chips. You dive into a yummy spaghetti (whole grain) and meat sauce dinner with your sweetheart as you watch an episode of *The Murdoch Mysteries*. You've just added another fifteen grams of protein to your daily total. Altogether, you've now had fifty grams of protein, falling far short of your goal of 72.5 since you weigh 145 pounds. You go to bed feeling happy and confident about your weight because you had no snacks today—just three healthy meals with whole grains, some fruit, and some vegetables. If you keep eating like this, you might feel a little sluggish as time goes on. Your clothes also don't fit the same way they did before. You are penalizing yourself in both a cosmetic and health sense.

Dr. Christine Gerbstadt, a spokesperson for the Academy of Nutrition and Dietetics, explains:

> There's a huge hormonal change that occurs around [the age of 50], particularly a decrease in estrogen and progesterone. However, with every passing year at this age—and it's much more significant in the 60s and

70s—there's a decrease in the basal metabolic rate or the energy required to maintain body weight. There's also an increased need for protein in the diet to maintain the same muscle mass as a younger woman.[3]

MINERALS AND VITAMINS

During menopause, levels of zinc, magnesium, and chromium fall. It is also common for women to fall short in daily iron intake, although the opposite may occur. For some women, increased iron during menopause poses a health threat.

Let's first look at the results of deficiencies in these four minerals, and how to overcome them, and then focus on the interesting menopausal challenge of too much iron.

Consult with your physician and/or nutritionist about how much you should be taking in each day, but keep in mind that absorption of the mineral is a complementary consideration to dosage. In trying to get the proper amounts of each, keep note of which other substances either increase or decrease absorption.

Zinc

The National Institutes of Health have determined that zinc deficiency is rare in the United States, even though the body doesn't store zinc. Omnivores should get plenty of zinc from animal protein. Vegans and

Table 9.1. Mineral Deficiencies Linked to Menopause

Deficiency	Some Key Results
Zinc	Decrease in muscle strength and endurance, reduced immune system function, less efficient metabolizing of nutrients, difficulty with wounds healing
Magnesium	Decrease to muscle tissue possibly resulting in cramps and muscle weakness, mental fogginess, weakened bones, fatigue, high blood pressure
Chromium	Depressed energy metabolism, with a high risk of diabetes
Iron	Decrease of oxygen transport throughout the body leading to abnormally low levels of red blood cells; loss of concentration and fatigue are two results

Table 9.2. Ways to Counter Mineral Deficiencies

Mineral	Absorption Increased By:	Absorption Decreased By:
Zinc	Amino acids	Calcium, iron, manganese, selenium, copper; whole grain foods and soy foods
Magnesium	Vitamin D (studies on this vary)	Too much, or not enough, calcium
Chromium	Amino acid chelates	Zinc, iron, and magnesium
Iron	Vitamin C	Calcium, magnesium, zinc, copper, chromium, and manganese; caffeinated beverages

vegetarians shouldn't have a problem either, though, because there is zinc in legumes, seeds like pumpkin and sesame, nuts, and dairy products.

But like every mineral that is derived from plants, the level is dependent on the quality of the soil in which the plants are grown. A great deal of our soil is very deficient in most, if not all, minerals. The only way to be certain if you are getting what you need, even with a diet that is theoretically high quality, is to be tested regularly for nutrients.

Magnesium

Every organ requires magnesium to function properly. Magnesium is necessary for the activation and function of seven hundred to eight hundred enzyme systems in the body. It catalyzes most of the chemical reactions in the body. It synthesizes protein; stabilizes RNA and DNA; transmits nerve signals; relaxes muscles, whereas calcium contracts muscles; and produces and transports ATP, your body's direct energy supply. And yet, ask your doctor about it and they may dismiss it as just a laxative!

In previous chapters, some menopause-specific benefits of magnesium have been noted, including some impressive anecdotal mentions of reductions in vasomotor symptoms when magnesium was increased. Focus on magnesium is warranted because the previous description of a magnesium deficiency just scratches the surface of what goes wrong when a mature woman lacks magnesium.

Before talking about the wonders of magnesium, however, it's important to point out that some studies suggest that magnesium absorption could be affected by calcium levels. This is one reason to discuss dosages with a nutritionist: you want to establish the right balance on a daily basis. Popping supplements and hoping for the best is generally not the way to go.

Magnesium is the fourth most abundant mineral in the body, with it serving key functions in myriad body processes. Magnesium deficiency can cause a long list of symptoms for menopausal women, some of which can be misinterpreted as direct results of the changes in hormone levels.

The very best, and most comprehensive, explanation of the importance of magnesium to every body—with particular focus on the body of a menopausal woman—comes from Dr. Carolyn Dean, whose insights contributed so much to this book. The title of Dean's book, *The Magnesium Miracle* (2017), suggests that the mineral is some kind of wonder drug. For most women, it may be close to it considering how many of us suffer from deficiencies. Even so, I'll repeat the advice that it's always best to start any supplementation practice by coordinating with your primary care physician and, hopefully, a nutritionist. (Medical doctors don't necessarily get nutrition courses in medical school.) Among Dean's top magnesium facts are these,[4] all of which are explored in depth in her book:

- Magnesium is necessary for the proper functioning of seven hundred to eight hundred enzyme systems in the body—that's why it can be implicated in scores of symptoms and dozens of health conditions.
- Most people (70 to 80 percent) are magnesium deficient.
- Calcium depletes magnesium in the body, and many people get too much calcium, either as supplements, in fortified foods, or in dairy products.
- Magnesium is very deficient in the soil and in the food supply, so it must be supplemented.
- Mitochondrial dysfunction is no longer a mystery. ATP energy molecules are made in the mitochondria. (See the section, "Principles of Energy.") Six of the eight steps in that cycle that produces ATP depend on magnesium.
- The definitive test that would tell you your magnesium levels, the ionized magnesium blood test, is not available to the public. A helpful but

less accurate test, magnesium red blood cell, must be used in conjunction with your clinical symptoms. The serum magnesium test is highly inaccurate, yet it is still the standard test used in hospitals, clinics, and most clinical trials—however, it doesn't even appear on an electrolyte panel.

- Magnesium deficiency is a major factor in chronic disease—diabetes, heart disease, high blood pressure, high cholesterol, migraines, irritable bowel syndrome, and heartburn. The drugs used to treat all these conditions deplete magnesium, often making symptoms worse.
- Telomeres, which are components of chromosomes, hold the key to aging, as does magnesium, which prevents telomeres from deteriorating.

To put it in lay terms, courtesy of a science-based UK-based website with a great deal of practical menopause advice called *A. Vogel*,

> Low levels of magnesium can interfere with your sleep. It can give you poor sleep pattern. It can cause low mood. It can even go as far as causing depression. It can cause muscle and joint aches and pains. It can cause fatigue. It can cause those horrible food cravings. It can also cause that kind of brain fog that we sometimes get. It can give us night cramps and restless leg. It can cause nausea. It can also cause low thyroid issues. It can cause high blood pressure. It can affect your hair and nails. It can make your hair really weak and it can cause split nails. And it can also trigger migraines and headaches.[5]

Sources of magnesium in food are so appealing that it's hard to imagine anyone not getting enough of this mineral. The short list of high-magnesium foods includes dark chocolate, avocado, nuts, legumes, flax and pumpkin seeds, salmon, bananas, and spinach. Even with the spinach, it sounds like a list of party food.

Chromium

Harvard Health Publishing titled one of its many informational papers for the public "Chromium: The Forgotten Mineral."

> It's one of the most common elements in the earth's crust and in seawater, but only tiny amounts are present in the human body. Its role in treating diabetes in animals was described in the 1950s. . . . It's wildly popular in

the United States as a supplement for weight loss, but it's not effective in that role. It's chromium: a forgotten nutrient that may finally get some respect because of new studies of chromium and heart disease, diabetes, and cholesterol.[6]

There are so many dietary sources of chromium that it's hard to imagine a deficiency; however, two staples of many American diets promote chromium loss: refined grains and simple sugars. So you may be eating your broccoli, having an apple a day, but face a reversal in your chromium levels because of your bagel for breakfast and mid-day soda.

Iron

If you're frequently tired, pale (women of color, take note: paleness can show up on the inside of the lower eyes and nails), experience shortness of breath, or have started suffering from headaches or heart palpitations, you might suspect iron deficiency. Go to your doctor. Iron deficiency can hit a woman at any age and can be triggered by health and lifestyle factors. Note that one of the substances that robs your body of iron is caffeinated beverages. Coffee might give you a hit of chromium, but it decreases your absorption of iron.

The flip side of the iron discussion is not too little, but too much. The authors of one study premised their research on the fact that estrogen levels drop in menopause, but an inverse change occurs in iron levels because the body is no longer losing so much iron in menstruation. Their suspicion was the abundance of iron could be a risk factor affecting the health of postmenopausal women. One of their speculations was that an iron overload could contribute to hot flashes. Research let them stand behind that speculation: "In contrast to iron deficiency leading to cold intolerance, an increase in iron might play a role in postmenopausal hot flashes."[7]

An overload of iron can also contribute to skin aging. Menopause has horrible effects on skin without this problem. It becomes thin, dry, and wrinkled due to changes in collagen and elastin content. The skin also has a diminished ability to retain fluids. Add to that the fact that

the human body has a limited capacity to remove excess iron; body iron is normally eliminated through the stool, urine, and exfoliation of epidermal cells. . . . When body iron storage increases, the skin is exposed to higher levels of iron, which may cause oxidative damage and skin aging during this process.[8]

As a menopausal woman, if you ever get the sense that you are in a no-win situation, this kind of research reinforces it. Fortunately, unless you have a serious overload, there are pleasant ways to reduce the iron in your body that won't change your lifestyle dramatically. Three of the simple ways offered by Livestrong.com[9] are:

- Drink tea or coffee along with your meals as often as possible. The tannins found in these beverages impair iron absorption.
- Avoid eating foods rich in iron; they will only make the problem worse. Limit your intake of red meat, which contains an easily absorbed form of iron, and sugar, which increases iron absorption. Iron supplements and foods fortified with iron are off limits.
- Consume eggs and fiber-rich foods, which hinder your body's ability to absorb iron. Some examples of high-fiber foods are raspberries, pears and apples with the skin, oatmeal, split peas, lentils, almonds, and sunflower seeds.

Vitamin A

Even more than minerals, in my experience as an athlete and fitness professional, I have found "vitamin abuse" a problem of women of all ages. My first exposure to it was in graduate school, when a friend who was an actress overdosed on vitamin A. She was taken to the hospital with an intense, unrelenting headache, arguing that the vitamin had cured her acne, so she would never stop taking it. Unlike water-soluble vitamins like C that you can wash out of your system, vitamin A is stored in the liver. I was once "cut off" at a juice bar for drinking too much carrot juice. The body converts beta carotene into vitamin A, and the "bartender" was told there was a health risk associated with binging on carrot juice!

Taking vitamin A supplements as part of a menopause health regimen is somewhat controversial. However, there are dietary sources of this vitamin, which can mitigate the effects of the loss of estrogen by helping to counter osteoporosis, heart disease, and urinary incontinence.

One source of controversy over vitamin A involves a study that linked increased levels of vitamin A with hip fractures in postmenopausal

women. In all fairness to the vitamin, however, the focus was on inges-
tion of what would be considered toxic amounts of vitamin A in supplement form.[10] It is still not clear how much non-dietary vitamin A could
lead to bone fracture risks.

For that reason, try to stick with dietary sources of vitamin A—orange and yellow fruits and vegetables.

Vitamin B-6

Of the eight B vitamins (1, 2, 3, 5, 6, 7, 12, and folic acid), the one that
menopausal women might focus on is 6, which helps make serotonin.
As chapter 4 described, serotonin is one of the "happy hormones" we
want to boost as we mature. To recap, fluctuating serotonin levels could
be an underlying cause of depressive episodes and feelings of anxiety in
menopause and after. Again, the reminder is that serotonin needs to be
in balance with dopamine to support a robust sex life.

If you are an omnivore, you should have no trouble sustaining B-6
levels through dietary means. Fish, pork, poultry, and beef liver and
other organ meats are good sources of the vitamin. Vegans can look to
brown rice, oatmeal, wheatgerm, and edamame. Vegetarians can add
eggs to the possible sources.

Vitamin D

You get this by playing, walking, or riding in a car with the sunshine
on you. As noted in Table 9.2, vitamin D promotes the absorption of
magnesium. This is part of its heroic role in reducing your risk of bone
fractures and bone pain.

In addition to sunlight, sources of vitamin D are fatty fish such as
salmon, as well as cheese and egg yolks. If you are a vegetarian or
vegan who keeps the curtains drawn, you have no choice but to take a
supplement.

Vitamin E

Vitamin E fights free radicals in the body, and it was recommended
to me decades ago by a peripheral vascular surgeon as something that
could counter inflammation. More recently, it was recommended as a

help in dealing with conditions common to menopause, most notably, depression. Consult with your doctor and nutritionist about whether to take a supplement. In the meantime, enjoy the almonds, hazelnuts, avocados, broccoli, shrimp, squash, and spinach that also deliver vitamin E.

THE FORCE OF MOVEMENT

Flexibility/Stretching

The July 16, 2018, headline read "Meet Olive, The 105-Year-old Who Can Still Touch Her Toes."[11] Olive clearly acknowledges a connection between flexibility and the QOL. The specific connection between stretching and QOL during menopause is not as obvious to most of us, however.

Advocates of various types of stretching regimens will provide anecdotal evidence of the way flexibility work improves QOL during menopause; however, there are also studies that document effects for randomized populations. One such study published in 2014 was designed to determine the efficacy of three non-hormonal therapies for improving menopause-related QOL in women with hot flashes and night sweats. The three therapies used over the twelve-week period were yoga, aerobic exercise, and omega-3 supplementation, with the 338 women who did the whole twelve-week program divided into three working groups plus a control group. These women were between the ages of forty and sixty-two years, with the average age being 54.7. Only one group had measurable improvement in menopausal QOL—those doing weekly ninety-minute yoga classes with daily at-home practice.[12] The yoga helped stabilize vasomotor symptoms, with an ancillary effect being better quality sleep.

Yoga scored well in a different 2014 study involving women aged forty-five to fifty-eight years, with four or more hot flashes per day on average. Again, the yoga classes were weekly ninety-minute sessions: "By week 10, women in the yoga group reported a decrease of approximately 66% in hot flash frequency."[13] There are different types of yoga, some of which might have the opposite effect on vasomotor symptoms because they are relatively strenuous. The yoga recommended as a therapeutic aid for symptoms involves primarily poses and stretching.

Forward folds from a standing position are a simple, very relaxing stretch that can have multiple benefits. Sending fresh oxygenated blood to the head is a calming move; as you do the fold, you also send blood to organs in the pelvic area. The increased blood also has the potential to elevate your sex drive. Drop your head and roll forward with your arms dangling. You can bend your knees a little, but only go down as far as it's comfortable. Raise yourself to an erect position slowly and then repeat the stretch a few times.

Stretching before bed can help you sleep better by moving tension out of the body and giving you an overall relaxed feeling. The National Center for Complementary and Integrative Medicine, which is part of the National Institutes of Health, surveyed more than thirty thousand households to determine reliance on and success with mind and body practices such as chiropractic and yoga and natural products such as echinacea and omega-3 fatty acids. Their findings indicated that over 55 percent of yoga users reported improved sleep and over 85 percent reported reduced stress.[14] Several yoga stretches/poses were specifically identified as helping to relieve tension and prepare the body for a restful sleep.[15] They include the following:

- The forward fold, described in the previous paragraph.
- Same stretch, but done bending only halfway and extending the arms in front of you.
- Lying on your back, arms outstretched to your side with your butt close to the wall and your legs upward, resting on the wall.
- If that doesn't work for you because putting your legs straight up creates too much strain, just rest your calves on the seat of a chair. Adjust yourself so your thighs are at a ninety-degree angle to your feet.

Strength/Resistance

Movements involving resistance are fundamental to preventing osteoporosis; stressing bones helps them stay strong. Doing some kind of resistance movement also slows down the inevitable sagging that leads to flopping arms and drooping breasts—and chores like stacking firewood, picking up a toddler, and carrying groceries all count as resistance movements.

If you have issues with the pelvic floor, then some resistance exercises must either be eased into or avoided entirely, at least until the pelvic floor weakness is addressed. Menopause and postmenopause years are a time when your pelvic floor can become your weakest link in your musculoskeletal structure. Take the following precautions recommended by PelvicFloorFirst.org if you have incontinence or other signs of problems, and then return to a more challenging routine after those problems have been resolved:

- Lighten your weights or resistance so that you don't feel pressure down on your pelvic floor as you move.
- Avoid holding your breath by exhaling with effort (e.g., when you pull, push, lift, or lower weights).
- Maintain good posture.
- Reduce the level of your abdominal muscle exercise programs, such as sit-ups.
- Reduce the depth of your squats and lunges; aim to keep your hips at a higher level than your knees.
- Choose supported positions (e.g., seated machines or sitting on a fit ball to use hand weights).
- Keep your legs closer together during exercise.
- Lift your pelvic floor before you move and relax afterwards. Notice how many reps you can do before your pelvic floor muscles tire. You may need to add some rests or reduce the number of reps that you do in a row, while your pelvic floor muscle fitness improves.[16]

The PelvicFloorFirst.org website provides a free, downloadable resource on pelvic floor–safe resistance exercises.[17]

Through the years, I've had many friends and acquaintances ask about my relatively toned mid-section and arms—particularly after I hit my sixties. When I tell them what I do, they invariable say, "I can't do that." The "that" is pushups. I get it: some people cannot do pushups because of physical limitations, including pelvic floor weakness. If you fall into that category, then download the above-referenced guide to alternate resistance exercises. If you don't have those physical limitations, before you join the chorus of "I can't do that," consider cosmetic outcomes: If you do just ten regulation pushups a day in succession, you've invested less than one minute in an exercise that can take years off your appearance and give you the ability to wear clothes you thought you would have to give to charity. Or, if you can't do them in succession, then take two or three minutes. This is not a timed exercise in front of a drill sergeant. The important thing is that you do them if you are able, not that you do them like an eighteen-year-old soldier.

Aside from improvement in appearance, why bother?

- Menopause is a time when so many things seem to be "going wrong" in the body that self-esteem can be eroded, and it's easy to have an encroaching sense that you've lost control. This is part of the shift in self-perception and attitude that profoundly affects the desire to be intimate. A pushup is a powerful and power-building move that can go a long way to restoring self-esteem.
- A pushup targets multiple muscle groups from shoulders to toes with special emphasis on the core, or mid-section, and upper body. In other words, you get a lot done with a single exercise.
- Because you target so many muscles in doing the exercise, your calorie burn is higher than with an exercise that targets just one muscle group. If one of your concerns is menopausal weight gain, every little metabolic boost helps.
- You can do pushups anywhere, anytime you're free, and wear almost anything you want. No need to go to a gym, use a mat, wear special clothes, make an appointment with a trainer, or find a partner.

A more fail-safe way to go to keep the upper body toned—because pushups can be not only daunting, but also dangerous if you don't do them properly—is to use exercise bands. Use a tension that makes you work; however, does not stress your muscles to the point of discomfort. Instructions on how to use them come with the bands, but it's wise to have at least one session with a personal trainer who can make sure you match the band tension to the exercise and that you do it in good form.

Coordination/Balance

With your bones and muscles perhaps not being all they used to be, it's especially important to prevent falls. If you have access to a recreation center or gym with classes in dance or yoga, try to attend at least once a week to do some focused work in the areas of coordination and balance. The practice of tai chi has proven to help coordination and relaxation. Pilates can also provide benefits in these areas, as well as strength-building moves.

If you are not someone who enjoys group workouts, then practice a few basic things at home like a single-leg stance or using an exercise band while lifting your legs forward and back and from side to side.

This entire chapter offered thoughts on modifying your lifestyle in little ways that will help you feel and look younger. If nothing else, do a few things to reduce stress, which research indicates can age a woman's chromosomes by ten years. In other words, stress ages you at the cellular level. With that thought in mind, here is a final suggestion from *Psychology Today* on a movement to reduce stress: "Sex is a great way to relieve stress. The benefits include release of endorphins and other hormones that elevate mood, and exercise, which itself is an effective stress reliever."[18]

Chapter Ten

Your Daughter's Menopause

On September 9, 2018, it was announced that TherapeuticsMD Inc. had earned a "buy" rating by brokerages covering the firm.[1] Who knew that was menopause news except those who stay current with hormone therapies? This is a company focused solely on women's health issues and their success to date could be seen as a trend toward greater investment in women's sexual health. Their contribution in a final phase of clinical trials is a product known as TX-001HR, "believed to be the first and only combination drug product candidate designed to replace the 17 ß-estradiol and progesterone hormones the ovary has nearly stopped producing."[2]

The day before, *Forbes* had a feature article on Mira Technology's "revolutionary" at-home hormone testing product, just approved by the US Food and Drug Administration (FDA).

> Any woman who has suffered from side effects of hormone replacement, or wrestled with the fatigue, weight gain, mood swings, diminished sex drive and insomnia of menopause, will understand the life changing possibilities of this product. No more trips to the OBGYN where your doctor throws up their hands when your hormone tests turn out normal. No suffering from hormone replacement therapies that often cause more problems than they fix. . . . While Mira doesn't solve the hormone replacement challenges for women, it does make it possible for women to see more accurately what hormones they need and how much and that can change everything.[3]

Again, the good news is not just that new menopause-related products are being reviewed, approved, and released, but also that the financial media find them important enough to cover.

Women's sexual health is finally serious news. Sometimes, it falls into the category of "odd" more than serious, but at least it's gaining prominence in terms of headlines. One of the 2018 stories that might be deemed "odd"—but could be a huge breakthrough for the orgasms of mature women—concerned the success of arousing women with an electric shock to the ankle.

It all began with University of Michigan researchers noticing that neuromodulation treatments (nerve stimulation therapy) for bladder dysfunction had the unexpected outcome of improving the woman's sexual function. Bladder dysfunction is commonly suffered by women going through menopause or who are postmenopausal. The researchers administered the nerve stimulation therapy once a week, with Dr. Tim Bruns identifying an interesting correlation that explained the outcome.

> In this particular treatment, a patient receives nerve stimulation therapy once a week to improve neural signaling and function in the muscles that control the bladder. . . . The nerves controlling the pelvic organs start out in the same location in the spinal cord and branch out.[4]

The electrodes providing the most stimulation to the pelvic organs happened to be located near the tibial nerve in the ankle. Brun's theory, which he investigated with a colleague in biomedical engineering, Dr. Nicholas Langhals, was that "the nerves that travel down to the foot overlap near the spinal cord with some of the nerves to the pelvic organs, leading to a possible overlap in synaptic routes."[5] Both of them wondered if any research involving nerve stimulation had ever been done with women struggling with sexual dysfunction who did *not* have bladder problems. They discovered nearly virgin research territory.

They focused new research efforts on rats and humans. The rats gave them a reason for optimism: "After 15 to 30 minutes, the rodents experienced a strong increase in vaginal blood flow."[6]

On to the humans. With the help of colleagues within the University of Michigan medical system, they recruited nine women with female sexual dysfunction who did not have bladder problems and engaged them in a pilot study. The results have led to the exciting, if ostensibly odd, articles about the sexual satisfaction associated with shocking a menopausal woman's ankles.

> A 53-year-old woman who got involved with the study after reporting to her gynecologist that she had difficulty achieving orgasm described the experience as "a bizarre pressure vibration sensation."[7]

She was not alone in her experience of unforeseen pleasure. Eight of the nine women in the pilot study reported improvement in arousal, lubrication, and orgasm. It was a small study group with an exceedingly high rate of success—hence the continued interest in zapping women's ankles.

In this final chapter, let's take a look at the most promising emerging and anticipated ways that menopause symptoms can be understood, mitigated, or eliminated, as well as the impacts of new developments on our intimate lives in the mature years. In addition to products and discoveries, we'll also explore medical and social trends that are helping to turn menopausal and postmenopausal years into sexual prime time. Interestingly, most of these new insights can be tucked into discussions of what we might call the "new myths of menopause"—the trending, well-hyped pieces of advice on how to manage menopause symptoms and reclaim diminished youth and vitality.

A NEW PATH TO HAPPY

In late summer of 2018, three key menopause-focused organizations finally came out with guidelines on assessment and treatment of perimenopausal depression. A team of doctors convened by the North American Menopause Society and the National Network of Depression Centers' Women and Mood Disorders Task Group, and endorsed by the International Menopause Society, crafted guidelines that were published concurrently in two journals, *Menopause* and *The Journal of Women's Health*.

One of the two co-lead authors, Dr. Pauline Maki, professor of psychology and psychiatry in the University of Illinois at Chicago College of Medicine, described perimenopause as "a window of vulnerability for the development of both depressive symptoms and major depressive episodes."[8] The significance of this may be simply that there was an official pronouncement of how at risk women are of depression during perimenopause and afterward, not directly because of the plunge in estrogen but because of effects of it. With that in mind, the authors said that contraceptives might reduce symptoms of depression a bit for perimenopausal women. But for women who have already gone through menopause, they made an unequivocal statement about *not* relying on hormone therapy for relief: "Estrogen therapy is not helpful in treating major depressive disorders in postmenopausal women."[9]

One of the opening points in the guidelines should alert every physician and every woman entering menopause to look for signs of trouble and not wait to take action: "The risk for depressive symptoms is increased in women during perimenopause even without a previous depression."[10] The authors caution that the other symptoms of menopause can put the focus on obvious physical issues, so the woman's depression may be overlooked and never be properly diagnosed.

Professor Laurie Santos is at the vanguard of medical professionals countering depression in creative, non-pharmaceutical ways. She taught the most popular class at Yale University when it debuted in 2017—in fact, it became the most popular class ever taught at Yale. First known as "PSYC 157: Psychology and the Good Life," it came to be known as the class on happiness. Because a whopping twelve hundred students took the inaugural course, she was able to share many research-based strategies for happiness in class. Ultimately, one out of four students at Yale took this class!

The fact that the students were young does not negate the potential value of the strategies for mature people, such as middle-aged women, who are fraught with family, professional, and social obligations—not to mention hormonal fluctuations. In fact, it's important to point out that the college experience of the late twentieth century was generally a much more fun-filled time than the college experience of this century. Middle-aged women facing a web of expectations from people around them, as they also experience major and confusion-causing shifts in hormone levels, may have much more in common with today's college students than in previous generations.

The "felt sense" exercise in chapter 8 will help inform you about your own baseline for happiness. It's part of assessing the affective facet of happiness, that is, your general mood, as well as how and where mood changes affect your body. Try maintaining that awareness as you experiment with the strategies Santos covered in her interview with host Ira Flatow for the popular National Public Radio program *Science Friday*:

- **Create time affluence.** Many of us deepen our anxiety and even put ourselves into a state of depression by trying to make time for everyone and everything. We create what Santos calls "time famine." The schedule that enables us to meet our obligations and feel as though we've accomplished what we had to robs us of the free time we need to be happy. "People who prioritize their time affluence are happier than those who don't, even when that comes at a cost of, say, how much money you make."[11]

  Santos took a risk on the day she was scheduled to teach the principles of time affluence: She cancelled class. The only ground rule that her students had that day was that the hour that had been freed up should be spent on something that would affect their well-being—not studying for a final or working on a term paper. Students hugged her, burst into tears, and threw themselves into the unfettered luxury of one hour with no obligations.

  For a woman experiencing both extreme mood swings and extreme demands on her time and attention, one free hour could be what releases a deep, aching pressure. The concentrated experience of time affluence could make the mood swings bearable and remind her—and everyone around her—that time to breathe, relax, and enjoy are essential to both mental and physical health.

  A couple can practice time affluence with a wink and a nod—or whatever signals availability in your relationship—and going to lunch, going for a walk, or going to bed for an hour. No expectations or agenda. Just pleasurable relaxed time together.

- **Make social connections.** The phrase "fake news" became hackneyed by 2017, before multiple articles and books focused on the topic to make us even more tired of those words. In terms of happiness strategies, a useful variation would be "fake conversation."

  Santos notes that the Yale students she encountered tended to spend more time alone than we might realize. Through social media, they are virtually connected, but they are not humanly connected. Instead of alleviating stress and engendering happiness the way spending time with a friend would, there is a paradox I would call "connection in isolation." People of any age can live this paradox with the myth of social connection through texting, phoning, and emailing. (When I'm embroiled in a book, I force myself to go to the grocery store so I can see girlfriends and have a conversation and a few hugs over the oranges. It's a mental health trip.) The extreme version of this is the experience of the Joaquin Phoenix character in *Her*, in which a lonely writer falls in love with an operating system who speaks to him with kindness and affection. Santos says, "The research suggests that you need to be there, in person, having these social connections. That's what matters."[12]

- **Pay it forward.** Research indicates that treating someone else with kindness and generosity boosts our mood. The phrase "pay it forward" was popularized by the 2000 film of the same name in which a boy ends up leading a movement to pay favors—not back, but forward—just choosing people at random for whom he does good deeds.

   Probably none of us would say "no" to the blatant opportunity to do a good deed for someone, like lending a hand when a person's crutch gives way and he falls on the sidewalk.

   But that's not the core message of "pay it forward." In that case, your radar needs to be attuned to ways to help your fellow human beings. For example, a friend of mine realized that her group of menopausal and postmenopausal (translate: sometimes difficult) friends probably needed a good laugh. Each of us got a note in the old-fashioned mail (US Postal Service) with a roster of jokes customized to our circumstances. There was no mistaking the level of love in those notes—and what she got back in terms of gratitude and loyalty is probably more than she gave us.

   "Paying it forward" is about the investment of your heart, not your bank account. No matter how many horrible things you are going through physically, your mind can help you power through and buoy you if you make this part of your life.

- **Go to sleep.** We all know that going to bed does not equate with going to sleep. After leaving social media behind, meditative practices can help us move toward the quality of sleep that helps counter anxiety and promote a feeling of well-being. But it is not just the quality of sleep that should concern us; it's quantity, too. If we don't get enough sleep to maintain mental health, we can induce psychosis!

• **Exercise daily.** According to the research Santos relied on for the course, a number of simple, health behaviors contributed to happiness: "A half hour of exercise every day is equivalent to the anti-depressant medication Zoloft."[13]

Implementing these happiness strategies requires altering habits. You want to install goals and cultivate habits that support well-being in a non-pharmaceutical, sustainable way. Assuming that a pill a day of hormone therapy will solve your issues of anxiety and/or depression is flawed thinking. In a best-case situation, a pill, injection, cream, or ovule is only a partial answer to what you're going through.

And now for the information that might really make you happy: Yale University has been offering Laurie Santos's course, now called "The Science of Well-Being" online for free.[14]

CONFRONTING THE "NEW MYTHS OF MENOPAUSE"

In the twenty-first century, we have seen what I deem the "new myths of menopause." These are health and lifestyle trends that might get play on the homepage of msn.com or be the subject of rabid bloggers. As popular as they might be, however, they can carry risks—or have no benefits at all. Here is a handful of them that can undermine your efforts to feel better if adopted without thought. At the same time, all of them have grains of medical wisdom embedded in them that *can* help you.

New myth #1: Probiotics do good things for you, and taking them is a safe bet.

For years, the hype on probiotics is that they will boost serotonin levels to counter depressive episodes, help adults shed pounds, strengthen a body's immune status—just about everything except guarantee everlasting life. Most recently, good news resulted from the first human study of the possible effects of probiotics on osteoporosis. For some women, probiotics have become a supplemental therapy to—or even a substitute for—some of the other treatments for their menopause symptoms. The name itself arouses feelings of trust and optimism, literally meaning "for life."

Massive numbers of people with disposable income clearly bought into the promises because the probiotics market was sized at over forty billion dollars in 2017 and is expected to nearly double by 2024.[15] Scientific data suggest it is not necessarily a good thing that the numbers are escalating so rapidly, however. In fact, they hint at the reality of probiotic abuse, confusion, and waste. Probiotics have a great deal of value, but don't deserve magic-potion status. A bit of background will point you toward facts on what they are, what to consider buying, what they can and can't do, and the potential harm of taking them.

The World Health Organization defines probiotics as live microorganisms that confer a beneficial effect when taken in adequate and appropriate amounts.[16] The persistent problem throughout this century so far has been the cloudy understanding of consumers of *which* live microorganisms are useful and *to whom* their beneficial effects might apply, as well as the definitions of "adequate" and "appropriate."

Benefits of probiotics are strain specific, so even two strains belonging to the same species do different things to and for the body. This is complicated: The human body supposedly has at least five hundred different probiotic strains.[17]

A common strain that most of us have heard of is *Lactobacillus acidophilus*, which is the strain associated with yogurt. It's naturally found in the mouth, intestines, and vagina. Purported benefits include reducing cholesterol, although one study found that it not only reduced "bad" cholesterol, but also "good" high-density lipoprotein cholesterol.[18] It is also credited with helping to prevent and reduce diarrhea, mitigating symptoms of irritable bowel syndrome, treating and preventing vaginal infections, promoting weight loss, averting symptoms of cold and flu, reducing allergy symptoms, preventing and mitigating symptoms of eczema, and generally improving gastrointestinal health.

The validity inherent in each of these benefit claims needs an explanation, because none can stand as an absolute. It's not as though you can reap all of these health benefits by having a daily cup of yogurt with "live active cultures." For example, the value of *L. acidophilus* in preventing and reducing diarrhea was documented in one study's collection of thirty-four trials; however, the results of those trials indicate that it generally worked much better with children than adults.[19] In addition, the conclusion is that its effectiveness depends on consuming it in combination with other probiotics. Regarding the usefulness of it in preventing and treating vaginal infections, *L. acidophilus* scored well in some studies and not so well in others. The most rousing endorsement we could give it is that it may be useful. And as a weight-loss supplement, some studies suggest taking *L. acidophilus* led to weight loss and some suggest it contributed to weight gain.[20]

In considering the variable nature of study results and caveats on effectiveness, keep in mind that *L. acidophilus* is just one strain out of hundreds, although we only see a dozen or so showing up in probiotic products. One product, on the expensive side, boasts "11 robust and potent strains." Another, on the inexpensive side, offers just one: *L. acidophilus*. In short, when someone swears by probiotics as part of a program of symptom mitigation and wellness, you are justified in wondering, "exactly what are you taking and how much?"

The positive study results related to osteoporosis concern a strain of lactic acid bacteria. Lactic acid is that substance produced in the muscle tissues during strenuous exercise that can build up and cause residual soreness. The downsides of the study are that it was small, with only ninety women, and that it involved only postmenopausal women aged seventy-five to eighty years. Nonetheless, it's worthwhile paying attention to the good news because it calls attention to the relationship between a single strain and a particular outcome rather than the randomness of "11 robust and potent strains."

One group took a twice-daily supplement of freeze-dried Lactobacillus reuteri, which is a strain of lactic acid bacteria. The other group was given a placebo. None of the women knew which group they had been assigned to. After a year, the bone density in the shins of all of the study participants was measured again. It turned out that the women taking the probiotic supplement experienced half as much bone loss during that year as did the women in the placebo group. And while that's a rather remarkable outcome, the authors of the study have a few words of caution. First, since this is the first human study of its kind, the data set is quite small. And second, the specific reasons behind the outcome of the study are not yet understood.

Still, the results are promising enough to ensure new and expanded studies. They add to both the interest in and the promise of the gut microbiome as a potential therapeutic target.[21]

The issue of "how much" is related to health risks in addition to health benefits. When the probiotic works as designed, the microorganisms

should go into the large intestine. Gastroenterologist Satish Rao is director of neurogastroenterology/motility at the Medical College of Georgia
and an experts on probiotics. His research documents that when probiotics migrate to the small intestine, the result can be disorienting brain
fogginess and rapid, significant belly bloating.[22] He also cautions that
there are hundreds of probiotic preparations on the market for which no
studies have been done, so the health benefits promoted on the labels are
questionable.

New myth #2: Natural products can help you and, at the least, will do no harm.

This feeds off the myth of probiotics being potentially helpful, but
never harmful.

The buzzwords "wellness" and "mindfulness" have led to attunement
to fitness and beauty products that have less to do with health than
they do with gullibility. *The Washington Post* reported the following in
September 2018:

> The market [for wellness products], estimated at $3.7 trillion in 2015 by the
> Global Wellness Institute, generates so many products and programs—salt
> rooms for increased mental clarity; rose quartz "eggs" for sexual health—
> that it's difficult for consumer and health watchdogs to keep up. Among
> the increasingly popular offerings that have drawn skepticism are vitamin
> patches, which not only (ostensibly) provide users with an influx of nutrients
> but are frequently marketed as a tool to kick-start a lifestyle makeover.[23]

Among the product offerings in this mix of "natural" remedies is the
"Menopause Night Relief" patch. The vitamin patch provides vitamin
D, niacin, riboflavin, thiamin, vitamin B9, selenium, magnesium, calcium, and a "complex" of other substances that have a mixed track record in terms of results, such as black cohosh and melatonin. Melatonin
isn't even a sleep aid in the customary sense; it's an aid to help regulate
the circadian rhythm so it's great for people traveling across time zones.
Black cohosh is used as an estrogen substitute and has gained substantial anecdotal, and even study support, over the years. The outcomes are
mixed, however. Some women have had great results in reducing the
symptoms of menopause. Nonetheless, the herb is unregulated by the
FDA so how much, how pure, and how often are critical questions in
determining whether you might try it.

Many social media reports sing the praises of "natural" products. Without the clinical studies providing data to document their proper dosage and identify the ideal population for success, your buying decision could be based on the praise of a woman whose genetics, lifestyle, environment, and diet are radically different from yours. It's a case of buyer beware.

New myth #3: Regular intense exercise triggers early menopause.

A Japanese study that made headline news in 2011 announced that women who do vigorous exercise or eat a heart-healthy diet reach menopause earlier than other women. It was based on self-reporting of thirty-one hundred premenopausal women over a ten-year period. News outlets blasted the message that exercise-hating thirty-somethings could use as an excuse to toss the spandex: "Women Who Exercise Often Hit Menopause Earlier."[24]

Many scientists were skeptical and stayed focused on an effort involving 107,275 women who were tracked through the Nurses' Health Study II, some of them joining the study as early as 1989. The conclusion announced in 2018 was the amount of physical activity women undertake has no bearing on the onset of menopause.

Dr. Elizabeth Bertone-Johnson, professor of epidemiology at the University of Massachusetts, directed the research. She said,

> Our study provides considerable information in helping us understand the relationship between activity and timing of menopause; this is because of its size, its focus on early menopause specifically, and because of its prospective design, which limited the likelihood of bias and allowed us to look at physical activity at different time periods.
>
> Several previous well-designed studies have found suggestions that more physical activity is associated with older age at menopause, but even in those studies the size of the effect was very small. Our results, in conjunction with other studies, provide substantial evidence that physical activity is not importantly associated with early menopause.[25]

In looking through all the data from the study, Bertone-Johnson pointed to environmental factors having a link to early menopause rather than exercise. Cigarette smoking and being underweight were two of the factors she singled out.

New myth #4: Your sex life can still be good, but it will never be as good as it was when you were young.

Throughout the earlier chapters in this book, a lot of rah-rah good news about sex after menopause has surfaced. Now it's time to be even more emphatic about the fact that the pleasure of sex after menopause can exceed anything you experienced when you were younger. The reasons for it are both psychological and physical.

In my early thirties, I was a bodybuilder and did quite well in regional competitions. I got accustomed to posing and strutting before large audiences in a very tiny, specially made, magenta bikini. It occurred to me that someday, I would no longer have a body that could get away with such exhibitionism, but that seemed decades away. The decades flew by. Suddenly, I was in my fifties and thinking it was more appropriate to wear a black one-piece suit, preferably with some compression in it. And shortly after that, it hit me: You'd better start loving this body you have because you'll never again have one that wins trophies. And so, I inadvertently learned one of the key points that Esther Perel teaches in her *Rekindling Desire* course: If you don't love your own body, then why would you invite anyone else to be next to you, close to you, inside you? As a corollary, when you do appreciate yourself, you are in a position to discover and maintain a connection to your "erotic self," in Perel's words.[26] That appreciation must include a physical dimension as intimate experiences always—somehow—involve the body.

Even women with spectacular bodies in their younger years are often plagued with the same insecurities that women with normal bodies have. At least one survey in the United Kingdom concluded that these insecurities begin to fade for many women once they hit forty and "by the time they reach their forties and fifties, women are more likely to feel 'happy,' 'confident' and 'secure.'"[27] A US study conducted at the University of Chicago found complementary results with a somewhat older population.[28] From a psychological perspective, therefore, mature women are generally better prepared to discover and enjoy their erotic self because they are more comfortable in their own skin.

The mechanisms of connecting to your erotic self are part of the magic of Perel's course. If you truly want to test my assertion that mature women have many advantages when it comes to creating the possibility of satisfying intimacy, I urge you to take her online course.

One thing you will discover is how to use your self-awareness and imagination to turn yourself on and turn yourself off.

Risk researcher and author Jim McCormick suggests one reason why mature women might choose to explore excitation in their lives in a way that they were unwilling to do previously. In his book, *The Power of Risk*, he includes the results of surveys about risk inclination he did with various populations. One firm conclusion is: "Women show increased risk inclination from their 40s to their 50s and on into their 60s."[29] He explains,

> This could be related to increased personal and professional options after the obligations to raise a family have been fulfilled. Some sociologists have suggested that women spend the first half of their lives tending to the needs of others, then, in some cases, spend the second half of their lives addressing more of their own needs.[30]

A 2013 study published in *The Journals of Gerontology* got a bit more specific about older women and risk-taking in terms of intimate encounters. While men typically took greater risks than women in many recreational situations throughout their lives (drinking, drug use, driving, sex, and so on), "gender differences reduced with age"[31]—and one of the specific references was to sexual activities.

On the physical side of the equation, it might seem odd to assert that mature women can have better sex, particularly since the early part of this book focused so much on the physically altering symptoms of menopause. Here's the paradox: Because we have more physical challenges related to having enjoyable sex, we can be more adept at having it. Our young ever-wet counterparts ostensibly don't have to do anything to create pleasurable circumstances—and so they don't. In contrast, we are more likely to know the difference between a silicone lube and a water-based one. We also might have a greater tendency to be more calculating about how, when, and where sex occurs because we're not going to put up with an overly air-conditioned room when we'd prefer making love on a sun-drenched terrace.

By the time you've hit menopause—at the latest—you should feel as though you've earned the right to have sublime pleasure. And by that time, you hopefully know enough about your body so that you can choreograph the occurrence of it.

Another critical element in transcendent intimacy is the trust we feel with our partner. Having the (hopefully) good fortune of years together,

we can learn to communicate about the how, when, and where that put
us on the path to erotic splendor.

New myth #5: Your doctor has all the answers on addressing menopause symptoms.

Physicians are just the beginning of solutions and opportunities. Without question, medical science in this century reflects astonishing progress. Due to their training and experience, physicians tend to have a
deep knowledge—of a few areas. Go to your doctor first, but don't go
only to your doctor.

Women of today have a wealth of resources and expertise that our
mothers did not. Physical therapists specializing in pelvic floor issues,
massage therapists with expertise in aromatherapy, and certified personal trainers accredited to work with older populations are just some of
the professionals who can help menopausal women alleviate symptoms
and improve their intimate lives.

Sometimes, of course, a medical doctor will add a channel of expertise to her education to give patients a more comprehensive clinical
experience. Carolyn Dean, author of *Menopause Naturally* and more
than thirty other books, features holistic remedies from a medical doctor
who is also a naturopath. Dean's groundbreaking work in understanding the value of magnesium to menopausal women has been cited in
this book. Dean takes a balanced approach that even those drawn to
the most mainstream, Western practices would find reasonable. Despite
the fact that *Menopause Naturally* was first published in 1999, Dean's
general advice in mitigating symptoms is surprising similar to the latest,
"forward-thinking" advice I heard from other experts:

- Menopausal symptoms are lessened in women who have a healthy
  diet, exercise regularly, and have a healthy outlook on life.
- Hypoglycemic symptoms are exacerbated by menopause and should
  be treated with a proper eating schedule and a low refined-carbohy-
  drate diet.
- There are dozens of natural remedies for menopause and the symptoms of menopause.
- Hormone replacement therapy may be necessary for some women;
  in this case, natural hormones can be used instead of synthetic ones.

- Each woman must study the options, take responsibility for her own health, and make her own decision on menopausal therapy. Then she must find a doctor who will work with her.[32]

The growing number of FDA-cleared products also signals tremendous hope for menopausal women. Researchers and clinicians have collaborated to bring us many of the vaginal moisturizing and rejuvenation technologies described in previous chapters. There are also affordable devices, sometimes covered by insurance, that can have a direct bearing on the quality of your intimate life.

One such device is the Yarlap, developed to reestablish pelvic floor muscle tone, which impacts daily life in multiple ways. Diminished control can come from muscle strain, often associated with childbirth and certain sports, especially activities with repetitive impact such as volleyball or the strain of lifting heavy weights.

As a medical device, Yarlap's purpose is to eliminate urinary incontinence by essentially doing your Kegel (pronounced *Kay*-gil) exercises for you. Programmable to deliver different intensities of pulse, depending on need and comfort, it stimulates the pelvic floor muscles. Three programs are aimed at building strength, and three deliver massage to relax the pelvic floor muscles.

Yarlap has also proven itself a useful tool for women looking to enhance sexual response. It should never fall into the classification of a "sex toy"; however, once a woman develops competence with it, it has clear value in its ability to enhance intimate experiences. Brent Reider, who developed the device—along with several other, FDA-cleared medical devices—notes that the work of two researchers figures prominently in the assessment of the value of Yarlap in the context of sexual satisfaction. They are Elisabeth Lloyd and Beverly Whipple. Lloyd boldly asserted in her book *The Case of the Female Orgasm* that human female orgasm has nothing to do with reproduction and she documented the mechanics of it. With her colleague John Perry, Beverly Whipple is primarily known as the researcher who confirmed the existence of the G spot in 1981 while doing research on female urinary incontinence.

Arnold Kegel, the American gynecologist who developed the exercises that bear his name, said, "Sexual feeling within the vagina is closely related to muscle tone, and can be improved through muscle education and resistive exercise."[33] Since the muscles that spasmodically contract in orgasm are those same pelvic floor muscles, it is a popular and accurate perception to associate pelvic floor muscle tone with sexual performance. The pathway to pelvic floor muscle control skills for sexual performance—the "Baltimore Grip," famously associated with Wallis Simpson, comes to mind—requires pelvic floor muscle tone and control.

Pelvic floor muscle tone can be regained at virtually any age, as one of the unsolicited endorsements Reider received helps to confirm:

Hilary (81):
I am a licensed healthcare professional that used Yarlap to treat my nocturia (leaking urine at night) over a few weeks. I noticed the pelvic floor muscle control from using Yarlap to treat my nocturia increased my sexual performance and expression. Love making was enthusiastically experienced again, and the improved flexibility facilitated sexual expression which I was not expecting at 81.[34]

A device like Yarlap removes the confusion for some women over how to do something that they've often been told is a simple clench-release exercise. A significant number of women who try to tone their pelvic floor muscles with Kegels find it difficult to determine if their pelvic muscle exercises have been performed correctly, even with help from a health care professional. In fact, the leading cause women do not return for the second visit to their health care professional for pelvic floor exercise—estimates as high as 70 percent never return—is they believe the Kegel exercises do not work or take too much time and concentration.

After extensive testing, the FDA cleared Yarlap with AutoKegel to address all of these issues, including the control problems suffered by women with severe muscle atrophy. The muscle re-education it promotes not only addresses bladder control, but also improves sexual performance and improves sexual expression.

There are competitive devices that purportedly help train the user in Kegel exercises, but a caution is in order about how they work: Anything that connects to your smartphone can potentially transmit information about you. The digital records of your use, progress, targets, and other personal matters might feed a stranger's database.

With the development of new technologies, grasp of nutritional and herbal sources of remedies, expansion of health care expertise, increased investment in women's sexual health, and shift in mindset about the right of women to experience pleasure, we can document the dawn of a new era for mature women. Women going into menopause thirty years from now will likely look back on the early twenty-first century as a pioneering time in terms of transforming menopause from a phase of inconvenience to a period of opportunity.

Here is a final thought from Yarlap inventor, Brent Reider:

If you are well-informed, you are less likely to be taken advantage of by a company, a purported healthcare professional, or anyone else offering answers. You are more likely to act in your self-interest in a positive way—for your benefit and those around you.[35]

Resources

Center for Erotic Intelligence (centerforeroticintelligence.org)—A global collective of scientists, doctors, researchers, therapists, sexologists, educators, and activists focused on the study and dissemination of information about human eroticism.

Esther Perel (www.estherperel.com)—Noted psychotherapist and relationship counselor offers podcasts, articles, and video courses such as "Rekindling Desire" to help improve the quality of intimate relationships.

Look Both Ways (www.lkbthwys.org)—A non-profit specializing in reproductive health education.

National Sleep Foundation (www.sleepfoundation.org)—Dedicated to improving health and well-being through sleep education and advocacy.

North American Menopause Society (www.menopause.org)—North America's leading non-profit organization dedicated to promoting the health and quality of life of all women during midlife and beyond through an understanding of menopause and healthy aging.

Pelvic Floor First (pelvicfloorfirst.org.au)—A service of the Continence Foundation of Australia that focuses on pelvic floor health.

The Welcomed Consensus (www.welcomed.com)—A community of instructors who teach techniques in communication and sensuality to access and develop sensual potential; they focus on female orgasm.

Women's Health Concern (www.womens-health-concern.org)—The patient arm of the British Menopause Society.

SELECTED BOOKS ON
MENOPAUSE AND INTIMACY

Allmen, Tara. *Menopause Confidential: A Doctor Reveals the Secrets to Thriving Through Midlife* (reprint edition). New York: HarperOne, 2017.

Boston Women's Health Book Collective, Judy Norsigian, and Vivian Pinn. *Our Bodies, Ourselves: Menopause*. New York: Touchstone, 2006.

Chapman, Gary. *The 5 Love Languages: The Secret to Love That Lasts*. Chicago: Northfield Publishing, 2015.

Dean, Carolyn. *The Magnesium Miracle* (revised edition). New York: Ballantine Books, 2017.

Faubion, Stephanie S. *The Menopause Solution: A Doctor's Guide to Relieving Hot Flashes, Enjoying Better Sex, Sleeping Well, Controlling Your Weight, and Being Happy!* Birmingham, AL: Oxmoor House Books, 2016.

Gottfried, Sara. *The Hormone Cure: Reclaim Balance, Sleep and Sex Drive; Lose Weight; Feel Focused, Vital, and Energized Naturally with the Gottfried Protocol* (revised edition). New York: Scribner, 2014.

Guntupalli, Saketh R., and Maryann Karinch. *Sex and Cancer: Intimacy, Romance, and Love After Diagnosis and Treatment*. Lanham, MD: Rowman & Littlefield, 2017.

Kantrowitz, Barbara. *The Menopause Book: The Complete Guide—Hormones, Hot Flashes, Health, Moods, Sleep, Sex* (revised edition). New York: Workman Publishing, 2018.

King, Lori Ann. *Come Back Strong: Balanced Wellness After Surgical Menopause*. Kingston, NY: Gunnison Press, 2018.

Lee, John R., and Virginia Hopkins. *What Your Doctor May Not Tell You About Menopause™: The Breakthrough Book on Natural Hormone Balance* (revised edition). New York: Grand Central Publishing, 2004.

Lloyd, Elizabeth. *The Case of the Female Orgasm: Bias in the Science of Evolution*. Cambridge: Harvard University Press, 2006.

Nagoski, Emily. *Come as You Are: The Surprising New Science that Will Transform Your Sex Life*. New York: Simon & Schuster, 2015.

Northrup, Christiane. *The Wisdom of Menopause: Creating Physical and Emotional Health During the Change* (revised edition). New York: Bantam, 2012.

Perel, Esther. *Mating in Captivity: Unlocking Erotic Intelligence* (reprint edition). New York: Harper Paperbacks, 2017.

Streicher, Lauren. *Sex Rx: Hormones, Health, and Your Best Sex Ever*. New York: Dey Street Books, 2014.

Williamson, Marianne. *The Age of Miracles: Embracing the New Midlife*. Carlsbad, CA: Hay House, Inc., 2009.

Notes

INTRODUCTION

1. Randi Hutter Epstein, MD, "The Menopausal Vagina Monologues," *New York Times*, September 3, 2018.

CHAPTER ONE

1. Rebecca C. Thurston, Linda J. Ewing, Carissa A. Low, Aimee J. Christie, and Michele D. Levine, "Behavioral Weight Loss for the Management of Menopausal Hot Flashes: A Pilot Study," *Menopause*, January 2015; 22(1); 59–65; https://www.ncbi.nlm.nih.gov/pmc/articles/PMC4270932/.

2. Carolyn Dean, *The Magnesium Miracle* (New York: Ballantine Books, 2017), p. 285.

3. Yvette Brazier, "Exercise Eases Hot Flashes during Menopause," *Medical News Today*, December 20, 2015; https://www.medicalnewstoday.com/articles/304295.php.

4. "Demystifying Perimenopausal Weight Gain," Women's Health Network; https://www.womenshealthnetwork.com/menopause-and-perimeno pause/demystifying-perimenopause-weight-gain.aspx.

5. Tianna Hicklin, "Molecular Ties Between Lack of Sleep and Weight Gain," NIH Research Matters, March 22, 2016; https://www.nih.gov/news events/nih-research-matters/molecular-ties-between-lack-sleep-weight-gain.

6. Ibid.

7. Pamela Peeke, "Oh, Do You Know the Muffin Top?" WebMD; https://www.webmd.com/menopause/features/oh-do-you-know-the-muffin-top#1.

8. M. Neale Weitzmann and Roberto Pacifici, "Estrogen Deficiency and Bone Loss: An Inflammatory Tale," *The Journal of Clinical Investigation*, May 1, 2006; 116(5); 1186–94; https://www.ncbi.nlm.nih.gov/pmc/articles/PMC1451218/.

9. Jill Seladi-Schulman, "What Is the Hypothalamus?" Healthline Newsletter, medically reviewed by Seunggu Han on March 1, 2018; https://www.healthline.com/human-body-maps/hypothalamus.

10. M. S. Exton, A. Bindert, T. Krüger, F. Scheller, U. Hartmann, and M. Schedlowski, "Cardiovascular and Endocrine Alterations after Masturbation-Induced Orgasm in Women," *Psychosomatic Medicine*, May–June 1999; 61(3); 280–89; https://www.ncbi.nlm.nih.gov/pubmed/10367606.

11. Kalyn Weber, "Why Women Should Care About Testosterone," *InsideTracker*, May 14, 2014; http://blog.insidetracker.com/why-women-should-care-about-testosterone.

12. "Estrogen and Women's Emotions," WebMD; https://www.webmd.com/women/guide/estrogen-and-womens-emotions#1.

13. Interview with Lori Ann King, August 13, 2018.

14. Ibid.

15. "Your Guide to Menopause," WebMD; https://www.webmd.com/menopause/guide/menopause-information#1.

16. Nanette Santoro, "Perimenopause: From Research to Practice," *Journal of Women's Health*, April 1, 2016; 25(4); 332–39; https://www.ncbi.nlm.nih.gov/pmc/articles/PMC4834516/.

CHAPTER TWO

1. Emmanuele A. Jannini, Nan Wise, Eleni Frangos, and Barry R. Komisaruk, "Peripheral and Central Neural Bases of Orgasm," *Textbook of Female Sexual Function and Dysfunction: Diagnosis and Treatment* (Wiley Online Library, April 17, 2018), pp. 179–95; https://onlinelibrary.wiley.com/doi/10.1002/9781119266136.ch13.

2. "The Brain on Menopause," BrainHQ; https://www.brainhq.com/brain-resources/brain-facts-myths/brain-on-menopause.

3. Victor W. Henderson, "Cognitive Changes After Menopause: Influence of Estrogen," *Clinical Obstetrics and Gynecology*, September 2008; 51(3): 618–26; https://www.ncbi.nlm.nih.gov/pmc/articles/PMC2637911/.

4. Barbara B. Sherwin and Victor W. Henderson, "Surgical versus natural menopause: Cognitive issues," *Menopause*, May–June 2007; Volume 14, Issue 3; 572–79; https://journals.lww.com/menopausejournal/Abstract/2007/14071/Surgical_versus_natural_menopause__cognitive.5.aspx.

5. Ibid.

6. "Burning Tongue," 34 Menopause Symptoms; https://www.34-meno pause-symptoms.com/burning-tongue.htm.

7. Zuzanna Ślebioda and Elżbieta Szponar, "Burning Mouth Syndrome— A Common Dental Problem in Perimenopausal Women," *Menopause Review* (*Przeglad Menopauzalny*), June 30, 2014; 13(3); 198–202; https://www.ncbi .nlm.nih.gov/pmc/articles/PMC4520363/.

8. https://www.menopausecentre.com.au/tingling-extremities/.

9. Nini Callan, Ellen S. Mitchell, Margaret M. Heitkemper, and Nancy, F. Woods, "Constipation and Diarrhea during the Menopause Transition and Early Postmenopause: Observations from the Seattle Midlife Women's Health Study," *Menopause*, June 2018; Volume 25, Issue 6; 615–24; https://journals .lww.com/menopausejournal/Abstract/2018/06000/Constipation_and_diar rhea_during_the_menopause.9.aspx.

10. Emmanuele A. Jannini, Nan Wise, Eleni Frangos, and Barry R. Komisaruk, "Peripheral and Central Neural Bases of Orgasm," *Textbook of Female Sexual Function and Dysfunction: Diagnosis and Treatment* (Wiley Online Library, April 17, 2018), pp. 181–82; https://onlinelibrary.wiley.com/ doi/10.1002/9781119266136.ch13.

11. Ibid., p. 182.

12. Mal Harrison, "The Internal Clitoris," Center for Erotic Intelligence, November 2011; http://centerforeroticintelligence.org/internal-clitoris/.

13. Interview with Beverly Whipple, July 21, 2018.

14. P. Richette, M. Corvol, and T. Bardin, "Estrogens, Cartilage, and Osteo-arthritis," *Joint Bone Spine*, August 2003; Volume 70, Issue 4; 257–62; https://www.sciencedirect.com/science/article/pii/S1297319X03000678? via%3Dihub.

15. https://www.mumsnet.com/Talk/menopause/2687724-Stiff-sore-feet -menopause-or-something-else.

16. Carolyn Dean, *The Magnesium Miracle* (New York: Ballantine Books, 2017), p. 343.

CHAPTER THREE

1. Gina Kolata, "Study Is Halted Over Rise Seen In Cancer Risk," *New York Times*, July 9, 2002.

2. S. A. Tsai, M. I. Stefanick, and R. S. Stafford, "Trends in Meno-pausal Hormone Therapy Use of US Office-Based Physicians, 2000–2009," *Menopause*, April 2011; Volume 18, Issue 4; 385–92; https://www.ncbi.nlm .nih.gov/pubmed/21127439.

3. "HRT: Benefits and Risks," Women's Health Concern, British Menopause Society, November 15, 2017; https://www.womens-health-concern.org/help-and-advice/factsheets/hrt-know-benefits-risks/.

4. Denise Grady, "Hormone Use Found to Raise Dementia Risk," *New York Times*, May 28, 2003.

5. Writing Group for the Women's Health Initiative Investigators, "Risks and Benefits of Estrogen Plus Progestin in Health Postmenopausal Women," *Journal of the American Medical Association*, July 17, 2002; Volume 288, Issue 3; 321.

6. James Clark, "A Critique of Women's Health Initiative Studies (2002–2006)," *Nuclear Receptor Signaling*, 2006; https://www.ncbi.nlm.nih.gov/pmc/articles/PMC1630688/.

7. Gina Kolata with Melody Petersen, "Hormone Replacement Study A Shock to the Medical System," *New York Times*, July 10, 2002; https://www.nytimes.com/2002/07/10/us/hormone-replacement-study-a-shock-to-the-medical-system.html.

8. Robert A. Wilson and Thelma A. Wilson, "The Fate of the Nontreated PostMenopausal Woman: A Plea for the Maintenance of Adequate Estrogen from Puberty to the Grave," *Journal of the American Geriatrics Society*, April 1963; 347–62; https://pdfs.semanticscholar.org/1d80/95259b0947c449a248bb018c480fc5aa7733.pdf.

9. Ibid., 357.

10. Ibid., 358.

11. Winifred Liu, "Continuous Estrogen Treatment in Women," *Journal of the American Medical Association*, 1965; Volume 192, Issue 4; 332–33; https://jamanetwork.com/journals/jama/article-abstract/655438.

12. Gina Kolata, "Study Is Halted Over Rise Seen In Cancer Risk," *New York Times*, July 9, 2002.

13. Ibid. "Hormone Replacement Therapy: Knowledge and Use in the United States," Centers for Disease Control and Prevention, United States Department of Health & Human Services, 2001; https://www.cdc.gov/nchs/data/misc/hrt_booklet.PDF.

14. John Ashby, "The First Synthetic Estrogen," Letter to the Editor, *Environmental Health Perspectives*, May 1998; Volume 106, Number 5; https://www.ncbi.nlm.nih.gov/pmc/articles/PMC1533096/pdf/envhper00528-0015.pdf.

15. "What Are Bioidentical Hormones?" Harvard Women's Health Watch, Harvard Health Publishing, Harvard Medical School, August 2006; https://www.health.harvard.edu/womens-health/what-are-bioidentical-hormones.

16. Ibid.

17. Interview with Dr. Rebecca Dunsmoor-Su, July 17, 2018.

18. "Hormone Therapy: Benefits & Risks," The Menopause Society; https://www.menopause.org/for-women/menopauseflashes/menopause-symptoms-and-treatments/hormone-therapy-benefits-risks.

19. All quotes and information taken from an interview with "Joan" on August 20, 2018.

20. Interview with Dr. Robert Wool, July 11, 2018.

21. T. B. Clarkson and S. E. Appt, "Controversies about HRT—Lessons from Monkey Models," *Maturitas*, May 2005; Volume 51, Issue 1; 64–74; https://www.ncbi.nlm.nih.gov/pubmed/15883111.

22. "Custom-Compounded Medications," Women's Health Research Institute, Northwestern University; http://menopause.northwestern.edu/content/custom-compounded-medications.

23. Interview with Dr. Rebecca Dunsmoor-Su, July 17, 2018.

24. Miranda Hitti, "Oprah and Bioidentical Hormones: FAQ: Oprah Is Talking About Bioidentical Hormones for Menopause; Experts Weigh In," WebMD, January 15, 2009; https://www.webmd.com/women/news/20090115/oprah-and -bioidentical-hormones-faq#1.

25. Shannon K. Laughlin-Tommaso, "Bioidentical Hormones: Are They Safer?" Mayo Clinic; https://www.mayoclinic.org/diseases-conditions/meno pause/expert-answers/bioidentical-hormones/faq-20058460.

26. K. Holtorf, "The Bioidentical Hormone Debate: Are Bioidentical Hormones (Estradiol, Estriol, and Progesterone) Safer or More Efficacious than Commonly Used Synthetic Versions in Hormone Replacement Therapy?" *Postgraduate Medicine*, January 2009; Volume 121, Issue 1; 73–85; https://www.ncbi.nlm.nih.gov/pubmed/19179815.

27. Lori Ann King, *Come Back Strong: Balanced Wellness After Surgical Menopause* (Kingston, KY: Gunnison Press, 2018), p. 10.

28. Ibid., p. 46.

29. Andrea Eisen, Jan Lubinski, Jacek Gronwald, Pal Moller, Henry T. Lynch, Jan Klijn, Charmaine Kim-Sing, Susan L. Neuhausen, Lucy Gilbert, Parviz Ghadirian Siranoush Manoukian, Gad Rennert, Eitan Friedman, Claudine Isaacs, Eliot Rosen, Barry Rosen, Mary Daly, Ping Sun, Steven A. Narod, and the Hereditary Breast Cancer Clinical Study Group, "Hormone Therapy and the Risk of Breast Cancer in BRCA1 Mutation Carriers," *Journal of the National Cancer Institute*, October 20018; Volume 100, Issue 19; 1361–67; https://academic.oup.com/jnci/article/100/19/1361/950472.

CHAPTER FOUR

1. Descriptions based on a quiz created for kids on the endocrine system called "9 glands of the endocrine system," by Quizlet, free online curated learning content created by publishers, educators, and organizations; https://quizlet .com/81714460/9-glands-of-the-endocrine-system-flash-cards/.

2. Knvul Sheikh, "MDMA Could be on the Market Legally by 2021," *Popular Science*, November 30, 2012; https://www.popsci.com/fda-just-approved -final-stage-mdma-drug-trials.

3. Sharon K. Farber, "Why We All Need to Touch and Be Touched," *Psychology Today*, September 11, 2013; https://www.psychologytoday.com/us/blog/the-mind-body-connection/201309/why-we-all-need-touch-and-be-touched.

4. Edward Tronick, L. B. Adamson, H. Als, and T. B. Brazelton, "Infant Emotions in Normal and Perturbed Interactions," Paper presented at the biennial meeting of the Society for Research in Child Development, Denver, Colorado, April 1975.

5. "Still Face Experiment: Dr. Edward Tronick," uploaded on November 30, 2009; https://www.youtube.com/watch?v=apzXGEbZht0.

6. Tara Parker-Pope, "Is Marriage Good for Your Health?" *New York Times Magazine*, April 14, 2010; https://www.nytimes.com/2010/04/18/magazine/18marriage-t.html?mtrref=www.google.com.

7. J. E. Graham, L. M. Christian, and J. K. Kiecolt-Glaser, "Marriage, Health, and Immune Function: A Review of Key Findings and the Role of Depression," in S. Beach and M. Wamboldt (eds.), *Relational Processes in Mental Health*, Volume 11 (Washington, DC: American Psychiatric Publishing, Inc., 2006).

8. Lynette L. Craft and Frank M. Perna, "The Benefits of Exercise for the Clinically Depressed," *The Primary Care Companion to the Journal of Clinical Psychiatry*, 2004; Volume 6, Issue 3; 104–11; https://www.ncbi.nlm.nih.gov/pmc/articles/PMC474733/.

9. "Microbes Help Produce Serotonin in the Gut," Caltech, April 9, 2015; http://www.caltech.edu/news/microbes-help-produce-serotonin-gut-46495.

10. Jessica M. Yano, Kristie Yu, Gregory P. Donaldson, Gauri G. Shastri, Phoebe Ann, Liang Ma, Cathryn R. Nagler, Rustem F. Ismagilov, Sarkis K. Mazmanian, and Elaine Y. Hsiao, "Indigenous Bacteria from the Gut Microbiota Regulate Host Serotonin Biosynthesis," *Cell*, April 9, 2015; Volume 161, Issue 2; 264–76; https://www.ncbi.nlm.nih.gov/pmc/articles/PMC4393509/.

11. "7 Foods That Could Boost Your Serotonin: The Serotonin Diet," Healthline, August 28, 2018; https://www.healthline.com/health/healthy-sleep/foods-that-could-boost-your-serotonin.

12. Simon N. Young, "How to Increase Serotonin in the Human Brain without Drugs," *Journal of Psychiatry & Neuroscience*, November 2007; Volume 32, Issue 6; 394–99; https://www.ncbi.nlm.nih.gov/pmc/articles/PMC2077351/.

13. James McIntosh, "What Is Serotonin and What Does It Do?" *Medical News Today*, February 2, 2018; https://www.medicalnewstoday.com/kc/serotonin-facts-232248.

14. Hari Shanker Sharma and Aruna Sharma, "Breakdown of the Blood-Brain Barrier in Stress Alters Cognitive Dysfunction and Induces Brain Pathology: New Perspectives for Neuroprotective Strategies," in Michael S. Ritsner (ed.), *Brain Protection in Schizophrenia, Mood, and Cognitive Disorders* (New York: Springer, 2010), p. 243.

15. Chris Stubbs, Lisa Mattingly, Steven A. Crawford, Elizabeth A. Wickersham, Jessica L. Brockhaus, and Laine H. McCarthy, "Do SSRIs and SNRIs Reduce the Frequency and/or Severity of Hot Flashes in Menopausal Women," *Journal of the Oklahoma State Medical Association*, May 2017; Volume 110, Issue 5; 272–74; https://www.ncbi.nlm.nih.gov/pmc/articles/ PMC5482277/.

16. Nurul Azmi M. Rappek, Hatta Sidi, Jaya Kumar, Sazlina Kamarazaman, Srijit Das, Ruziana Masiran, Najwa Baharuddin, and Muhammad Hizri Hatta, "Serotonin Selective Reuptake Inhibitors (SSRIs) and Female Sexual Dysfunction (FSD): Hypothesis on its Association and Options of Treatment," *Current Drug Targets*, September 2018; Volume 19, Issue 12; 1352–58; https://www .ingentaconnect.com/contentone/ben/cdt/2018/00000019/00000012/art00003.

17. T. W. Kjaer, C. Bertelsen, P. Piccini, et al., "Increased Dopamine Tone during Meditation-Induced Change of Consciousness," *Brain Research Cognitive Brain Research,* 2002; Volume 13; 255–59.

18. Foods such as those listed, with the exception of fiber, contain the amino acid tryptophan; serotonin is synthesized from tryptophan.

19. M. R. Melis and A. Argiolas, "Dopamine and Sexual Behavior," *Neuroscience & Biobehavioral Reviews*, Spring 1995; Volume 19, Issue 1; 19–38; https://www.ncbi.nlm.nih.gov/pubmed/7770195.

20. Ibid.

21. Erin Brodwin, "The FDA Has Just Backed a Drug to Improve Female Sex Drive," *Business Insider*, June 5, 2015; https://www.sciencealert.com/ here-s-how-the-new-fda-backed-female-libido-pill-works.

22. J. A. Simon, S. A. Kingsberg, B. Shumel, V. Hanes, M. Garcia Jr., and M. Sand, "Efficacy and Safety of Flibanserin in Postmenopausal Women with Hypoactive Sexual Desire Disorder: Results of the SNOWDROP Trial," *Menopause*, June 2014; Volume 21, Issue 6; 633–40; https://www.ncbi.nlm.nih.gov/ pubmed/24281236.

23. Susan G. Kornstein, James A. Simon, Stuart C. Apfel, James Yuan, Krista A. Barbour, and Robert Kissling, "Effect of Flibanserin Treatment on Body Weight in Premenopausal and Postmenopausal Women with Hypoactive Sexual Desire Disorder: A Post Hoc Analysis," *Journal of Women's Health*, November 1, 2017; Volume 26, Issue 11; 1161–68; https://www.ncbi.nlm.nih .gov/pmc/articles/PMC5695746/.

24. Lizette Borreli, "Dopamine Diet: Naturally Control Hunger Cravings and Boost Weight Loss," *Medical Daily*, August 14, 2013; https://www.medi caldaily.com/dopamine-diet-naturally-control-hunger-cravings-and-boost -weight-loss-251265.

25. Andrew Weil, MD, "6 Simple Ways To Improve Low Mood"; https:// www.drweil.com/blog/spontaneous-happiness/6-simple-ways-to-improve -low-mood/.

26. Ibid.

CHAPTER FIVE

1. Interview with Dr. Betsy Cairo on August 25, 2018.

2. Carl Zimmer, "The Brain: Where Does Sex Live in the Brain? From Top to Bottom," *Discover*, October 2009; http://discovermagazine.com/2009/oct/10-where-does-sex-live-in-brain-from-top-to-bottom.

3. Ibid.

4. Ibid.

5. Interview with Dr. Betsy Cairo on August 25, 2018.

6. Emily Nagoski, "The Truth about Unwanted Arousal," TED2018, April 2018; https://www.ted.com/talks/emily_nagoski_the_truth_about_un wanted_arousal.

7. Jordan Gaines Lewis, "Smells Ring Bells: How Smell Triggers Memories and Emotions," *Psychology Today*, January 12, 2015; https://www.psy chologytoday.com/us/blog/brain-babble/201501/smells-ring-bells-how-smell -triggers-memories-and-emotions.

8. Joshua Foer, "Feats of Memory Anyone Can Do," TED2012, February 2012; https://www.ted.com/talks/joshua_foer_feats_of_memory_anyone_can_do.

9. Esther Perel, "Rekindling Desire: Defining Desire," uploaded August 31, 2018; https://vimeo.com/287516689/d238cceab9.

10. Susan Krauss Whitbourne, "Finding Joy in the Sexless Marriage: Why Do Relationships Become Sexless and How Do Couples Cope?" *Psychology Today*, February 22, 2014; https://www.psychologytoday.com/us/blog/fulfillment-any-age/201402/finding-joy-in-the-sexless-marriage.

11. Ibid.

12. David Brooks, "The Heart Grows Smarter," *New York Times*, November 5, 2012; https://www.nytimes.com/2012/11/06/opinion/brooks-the-heart -grows-smarter.html.

13. Ibid.

14. Peggy Orenstein, "Saving Our Daughters from an Army of Princesses," *All Things Considered*, National Public Radio; http://www.npr .org/2011/02/05/133471639/saving-our-daughters-from-an-army-of-princesses.

15. Peggy Orenstein, *Cinderella Ate My Daughter: Dispatches from the Front Lines of the New Girlie-Girl Culture* (New York: Harper, 2011), p. 2.

CHAPTER SIX

1. Eve Ensler, *The Vagina Monologues* (New York: Villard, 2007), p. 124.

2. Email from Lori Ann King, August 2, 2018.

3. Interview with Alyssa Dweck, July 10, 2018.

4. C. Lentza-Rizos and E. J. Avramides, "Pesticide Residues in Olive Oil," *Reviews of Environmental and Contamination Toxicology*, 1995; Volume 141; 111–34; https://www.ncbi.nlm.nih.gov/pubmed/7886254.

5. Deborah Grady, "Management of Menopausal Symptoms," *New England Journal of Medicine*, November 30, 2006; Volume 355; 2338–347; https://www.nejm.org/doi/full/10.1056/NEJMcp054015.

6. "Replens Review: How Safe and Effective Is This Product?" *Consumer Health Digest*; https://www.consumerhealthdigest.com/female-enhancement-products/replens.html.

7. Interview with Alyssa Dweck, July 10, 2018.

8. Azam Jokar, Tayebe Davari, Nasrin Asadi, Fateme Ahmadi, and Sedighe Foruhari, "Comparison of the Hyaluronic Acid Vaginal Cream and Conjugated Estrogen Used in Treatment of Vaginal Atrophy of Menopause Women: A Randomized Controlled Clinical Trial," *International Journal of Community Based Nurse Midwifery*, 2016; Volume 4, Issue 1; 69–78; https://www.ncbi.nlm.nih.gov/pmc/articles/PMC4709811/.

9. https://www.premarinvaginalcream.com/.

10. Korin Miller, "Yup, Laser Vaginal Tightening Is A Thing. Here's What It's All About," *Glamour*, March 28, 2016; https://www.glamour.com/story/yup-laser-vaginal-tightening-i.

11. Cheryl Karcher and Neil Sadick, "Vaginal Rejuvenation using Energy-Based Devices," *International Journal of Women's Dermatology*, September 2016; Volume 2, Issue 3; 85–88; https://www.ncbi.nlm.nih.gov/pmc/articles/PMC5418869/.

12. "Six Scientific Publications Confirm the Effectiveness and Safety Of Co2 Fractional Laser Treatment, Now Approved Worldwide," MonaLisa Touch website, posted April 30, 2015; http://www.monalisatouch.com/sure-and-effective/.

13. Interview with Rebecca Dunsmoor-Su, July 17, 2018.

14. Salil Khandwala, "MonaLisa Touch Study," Michigan Institution of Women's Health PC, Clinical Trials.gov, posted November 6, 2017, and updated December 5, 2017; U.S. National Library of Medicine; https://clinicaltrials.gov/ct2/show/NCT03331328.

15. Ibid.

16. Ibid.

17. Interview with Rebecca Dunsmoor-Su, July 17, 2018.

18. Paul W. Andrews, Susan G. Kornstein, Lisa J. Halberstadt, Charles O. Gardner, and Michael C. Neale, "Blue Again: Perturbational Effects of Antidepressants Suggest Monoaminergic Homeostasis in Major Depression," *Frontiers of Psychology*, July 7, 2011; https://www.frontiersin.org/articles/10.3389/fpsyg.2011.00159/full.

19. "Important Safety Information," Brisdelle website; https://brisdelle.com/.

20. "Natural Remedies for Hot Flashes," Menopause Society; https://www.menopause.org/for-women/menopauseflashes/menopause-symptoms-and-treatments/natural-remedies-for-hot-flashes.

21. Ibid.

22. Atieh Hajirahimkhan, Birgit M. Dietz, and Judy L. Bolton, "Botanical Modulation of Menopausal Symptoms: Mechanisms of Action?" *Planta Medica*, May 2013; Volume 79, Issue 7; 538–53; https://www.ncbi.nlm.nih.gov/pmc/articles/PMC3800090/.

23. Marya Ahsan and Ayaz Khurram Mallick, "The Effect of Soy Isoflavones on the Menopause Rating Scale Scoring in Perimenopausal and Postmenopausal Women: A Pilot Study," *Journal of Clinical & Diagnostic Research*, September 2017; Volume 11, Issue 9; FC13–FC16; https://www.ncbi.nlm.nih.gov/pmc/articles/PMC5713750/.

24. Samira Ziaei and Reginald Halaby, "Dietary Isoflavones and Breast Cancer Risk," *Medicines*, June 2017; Volume 4, Issue 2; 18; https://www.ncbi.nlm.nih.gov/pmc/articles/PMC5590054/.

25. Didem Sunay, Muruvvet Ozdiken, Huseyin Arslan, Ali Seven, and Yalcin Aral, "The Effect of Acupuncture on Postmenopausal Symptoms and Reproductive Hormones: A Sham Controlled Clinical Trial," *BMJ Journals*, 2011; Volume 29, Issue 1; 27–31; https://journals.sagepub.com/doi/pdf/10.1136/aim.2010.003285.

26. Amanda Macmillan, "Got Hot Flashes? Acupuncture May Offer Relief, Study Finds," *Health*, September 30, 2016; https://www.health.com/menopause/hot-flashes-menopause-acupuncture.

27. Interview with Brian Boitano, 1999, as reported in *Lessons from the Edge* (Simon & Schuster, 2000); all rights reverted to author.

28. Michael Finkel, citing Steven Lockley in "Want To Fall Asleep? Read This Story," *National Geographic*, August 2018, p. 66.

29. Joyce Walsleben, "How Is Sleep Affected by Perimenopause, Menopause, and Post-Menopause?" National Sleep Foundation; https://sleepfoundation.org/ask-the-expert/menopause-and-insomnia.

30. Ronald L. Kotler and Maryann Karinch, *365 Ways to Get a Good Night's Sleep* (Avon, MA: AdamsMedia, 2009), pp. 175–76.

31. Kazem M. Azadzoi and Mike B. Siroky, "Neurologic Factors in Female Sexual Function and Dysfunction," *Korean Journal of Urology*, July 2010; Volume 51, Issue 7; 443–49; https://www.ncbi.nlm.nih.gov/pmc/articles/PMC2907491/.

CHAPTER SEVEN

1. https://coad7404.files.wordpress.com/2014/06/extragenitalmatrix1.pdf.

2. Linda Weiner and Constance Avery-Clark, "Sensate Focus: Clarifying the Masters and Johnson's Model," *Sexual and Relationship Therapy*, 2014; Volume 29, Issue 3.

3. https://www3.nd.edu/~pmtrc/Handouts/Sensate_Focus.pdf.

4. William H. Masters, Virginia E. Johnson, and Robert C. Kolodny, *Heterosexuality* (New York: HarperCollins, 1994), p. 29.

5. https://health.cornell.edu/sites/health/files/pdf-library/sensate-focus.pdf.

6. Elizabeth Gilbert, *Eat, Pray, Love: One Woman's Search for Everything Across Italy, India, and Indonesia* (New York: Riverhead Books, 2007), p. 88.

7. Orson Scott Card, *Children of the Mind* (New York: Tor Science Fiction, 1997), p. 221.

8. Melissa Willets, "Shhh . . . 9 Secrets Women Keep From Men," *PopSugar*, July 31, 2018; http://www.msn.com/en-us/lifestyle/family-relationships/shhh-9-secrets-women-keep-from-men/ss-BBLjtYk?li=BBnb7Kz.

9. Yvonne Wray, "Help for Menopause: How I Got Relief and Gained Happiness," *The Welcomed Consensus*; https://www.welcomed.com/blog/help-for-menopause-got-relief-gained-happiness/.

10. Interview with Yvonne Wray of *The Welcomed Consensus*, August 6, 2018.

11. Yvonne Wray, "Down for the Count," with additional contributions and permissions from Yvonne Wray; https//www.welcomed.com/blog/what-do-hot-flashes-feel-like/.

12. Ibid.

13. Ibid.

14. James A. Coan, Hillary S. Schaefer, and Richard J. Davidson, "Lending a Hand: Social Regulation of the Neural Response to Threat," *Psychological Science*, December 1, 2006; http://journals.sagepub.com/doi/abs/10.1111/j.1467-9280.2006.01832.x.

15. Brené Brown, "Listening to Shame," TED2012, March 2012; https://www.ted.com/talks/brene_brown_listening_to_shame.

16. Gary Chapman, *The 5 Love Languages: The Secret to Love That Lasts* (Chicago, IL: Northfield Publishing, reprinted 2015).

CHAPTER EIGHT

1. Dena Bunis, "Two-Thirds of Older Adults Are Interested in Sex, Poll Says," *AARP*, May 3, 2018; https://www.aarp.org/health/healthy-living/info2018/older-sex-sexual-health-survey.html.

2. Ibid.

3. Sarah Jio, "The Truth about Sex after Menopause," *Woman's Day*, October 27, 2009; https://www.womansday.com/relationships/sex-tips/a4354/the-truth-about-sex-after-menopause-99603/.

4. Esther Perel, "Rekindling Desire" (Proprietary material, accessible through EstherPerel.com).

5. Larry Senn, "Why Is Gratitude At the Top Of the Mood Elevator?" July 1, 2017; https://themoodelevator.com/mood-elevator-tips/why-is-gratitude-at-the-top-of-the-mood-elevator/.

6. http://www.merriam-webster.com/dictionary/love.

7. Esther Perel, "Rekindling Desire" (Proprietary material, accessible through EstherPerel.com).

8. Winona Dimeo-Ediger, "Why Women Put Others' Happiness Before Their Own," *Ravishly*, June 25, 2015; https://ravishly.com/2015/06/25/why-women-put-others%E2%80%99-happiness-their-own.

9. Interview with Jennifer A. Skyler, September 14, 2016.

10. "30 Day Pleasure Challenge," https://www.welcomed.com/wp-content/uploads/2018/05/30-Day-Challenge-for-Pleasure-Calendar.pdf.

11. Saketh Guntupalli and Maryann Karinch, *Sex and Cancer* (Lanham, MD: Rowman & Littlefield, 2017), pp. 135–36.

12. Interview with Jennifer A. Skyler, September 14, 2016.

CHAPTER NINE

1. Interview with Scott Connelly for *Lessons from the Edge* (New York: Simon & Schuster, 2000), pp. 81–82.

2. C. Castaneda, J. M. Charnley, W. J. Evans, and M. C. Crim, "Elderly Women Accommodate to a Low-protein Diet with Losses of Body Cell Mass, Muscle Function, and Immune Response," *The American Journal of Clinical Nutrition*, July 1995; Volume 62, Issue 1; 30–39; https://www.ncbi.nlm.nih.gov/pubmed/7598064.

3. Christine Gerbstadt as interviewed by Lenora Dannelke for "Flourishing at Age 50 and Beyond—A Healthful Diet Plus Physical Activity Are Essential," *Today's Dietitian*, August 2012; https://www.todaysdietitian.com/newarchives/080112p58.shtml.

4. Paraphrased from Carolyn Dean, *The Magnesium Miracle, 2017 Revised and Updated Edition* (New York: Ballantine Books, 2017), pp. xxi–xxii.

5. Eileen Durward, "A. Vogel Talks Menopause: Why You Need Magnesium during Menopause," October 3, 2016; https://www.avogel.co.uk/health/menopause/videos/why-you-need-magnesium-during-menopause/.

6. "Chromium: The Forgotten Mineral," *Harvard Health Publishing*, January 2007; https://www.health.harvard.edu/newsletter_article/chromium-the-forgotten-mineral.

7. Jinlong Jian, Edward Pelle, and Xi Huang, "Iron and Menopause: Does Increased Iron Affect the Health of Postmenopausal Women?" *Antioxidants & Redox Signaling*, December 2009; Volume 11, Issue 12; 2939–43; https://www.ncbi.nlm.nih.gov/pmc/articles/PMC2821138/.

8. Ibid.

9. Joshua McCarron, "How To Get Rid of Excess Iron In the Human Body," *Livestrong.com*, October 3, 2017; https://www.livestrong.com/article/185197-how-to-get-rid-of-excess-iron-in-the-human-body/.

10. D. Feskanich, V. Singh, W. C. Willett, and G. A. Colditz, "Vitamin A Intake and Hip Fractures among Postmenopausal Women," *Journal of the American Medical Association*, January 2002; Volume 287, Issue 1; 47–54; https://www.ncbi.nlm.nih.gov/pubmed/11754708.

11. Miranda Larbi, "Meet Olive, The 105-Year-Old Who Can Still Touch Her Toes," *Metro*, July 16, 2018; https://metro.co.uk/2018/07/16/meet-olive-105-year-old-can-still-touch-toes-7719876/.

12. Susan D. Reed, K. A. Guthrie, K. M. Newton, et al., "Menopausal Quality of Life: A RCT of Yoga, Exercise and Omega-3 Supplements," *American Journal of Obstetrics and Gynecology*, March 2014; Volume 210, Issue 3; 244. e1–244.e11; https://www.ncbi.nlm.nih.gov/pmc/articles/PMC3976276/.

13. Nancy E. Avis, Claudine Legault, Gregory Russell, Kathryn Weaver, and Suzanne C. Danhauer, "A Pilot Study of Integral Yoga for Menopausal Hot Flashes," *Menopause*, August 2014; Volume 21, Issue 8; 846–54; https://www.ncbi.nlm.nih.gov/pmc/articles/PMC4110168/.

14. "Use of Complementary Health Approaches in the U.S." National Health Interview Survey, National Center for Complementary and Integrative Health, National Institutes of Health, 2015; https://nccih.nih.gov/research/statistics/NHIS/2012/wellness?nav=chat.

15. Marlynn Wei, "Yoga for Better Sleep," *Harvard Health Publishing*, December 4, 2015; https://www.health.harvard.edu/blog/8753-201512048753.

16. "The Pelvic Floor and Resistance Exercises"; http://www.pelvicfloorfirst.org.au/pages/pelvic-floor-safe-resistance-exercises.html.

17. http://www.pelvicfloorfirst.org.au/data/files/The_pelvic_floor_and_resistance_exercises.pdf.

18. Andrew Goliszek, "The Stress-Sex Connection," *Psychology Today*, December 22, 2014; https://www.psychologytoday.com/us/blog/how-the-mind-heals-the-body/201412/the-stress-sex-connection.

CHAPTER TEN

1. "TherapeuticsMD Inc (TXMD) Given Average Rating of 'Buy' By Brokerages," *American Banking and Market News*, September 9, 2018.

2. TX-001HR (Oral Estradiol & Progesterone), Research & Development, TherapeuticsMD, Inc.; https://www.therapeuticsmd.com/research/tx001hr.

3. Western Bonime, "Mira's Biotechnology Brings Hope for Fertility and Menopause," *Forbes*, September 8, 2018.

4. Dr. Tim Bruns, as quoted by Kelly Malcom, "Simple Nerve Stimulation May Improve Sexual Response in Women," HealthLab (University of Michigan), September 6, 2018; https://labblog.uofmhealth.org/body-work/simple-nerve-stimulation-may-improve-sexual-response-women.

5. Ibid.

6. Ibid.

7. Ibid.

8. "Very First Recommendations to Assess and Treat Perimenopausal Depression," *Medindia*, September 7, 2018.

9. Ibid.

10. Ibid.

11. Laurie Santos, as interviewed by Ira Flatow for "What Makes Your Brain Happy?" *Science Friday*, WNYC/NPR, July 13, 2018; https://www.sciencefriday.com/segments/what-makes-your-brain-happy/.

12. Ibid.

13. Ibid.

14. https://www.coursera.org/learn/the-science-of-well-being.

15. Industry Report, Global Market Insights; https://www.gminsights.com/industry-analysis/probiotics-market.

16. "Evaluation of Health and Nutritional Properties of Powder Milk and Live Lactic Acid Bacteria," Food and Agriculture Organization of the United Nations and World Health Organization Expert Consultation Report, Cordoba, Argentina (2001), pp. 1–34.

17. "Top 15 Most Researched Probiotic Strains," *Probiotics.org*; http://probiotics.org/strains/.

18. Ruairi Robertson, "9 Ways Lactobacillus Acidophilus Can Benefit Your Health," *Healthline*, June 14, 2017; https://www.healthline.com/nutrition/lactobacillus-acidophilus.

19. S. Sazawal, G. Hiremath, U. Dhingra, P. Malik, S. Deb, and R. E. Black, "Efficacy of Probiotics in Prevention of Acute Diarrhoea: A Meta-Analysis of Masked, Randomised, Placebo-Controlled Trials," *The Lancet Infectious Diseases*, June 2006; Volume 6, Issue 6; 374–82; https://www.ncbi.nlm.nih.gov/pubmed/16728323.

20. M. Million, E. Angelakis, M. Paul, F. Armougom, L. Leibovici, and D. Raoult, "Comparative Meta-Analysis of the Effect of Lactobacillus Species on Weight Gain in Humans and Animals," *Microbial Pathogenesis*, August 2012; Volume 53, Issue 2; 100–08; https://www.ncbi.nlm.nih.gov/pubmed/22634320.

21. Eve Glazier and Elizabeth Ko, "Ask the Doctors; Study Reveals Probiotics May Slow Osteoporosis," *Brattleboro Reformer (Vermont)*, September 3, 2018.

22. Satish S. C. Rao, "Probiotic Use is a Link between Brain Fogginess, Severe Bloating," *Science Daily*, August 6, 2018; https://www.sciencedaily.com/releases/2018/08/180806095213.htm.

23. Sarah Baird, "A Sticky Situation?" *The Washington Post*, September 6, 2018.

24. "Women Who Exercise Often Hit Menopause Earlier," *Reuters*, October 12, 2011; http://www.foxnews.com/health/2011/10/12/women-who-exercise-often-hit-menopause-earlier.html.

25. "Exercise is Unrelated to Risk of Early Menopause," *Indian Health Care News*, September 8, 2018.

26. Esther Perel, "Rekindling Desire" (Proprietary material, accesible through EstherPerel.com).

27. "REVEALED: Women Become Comfortable With Themselves at THIS Age," *Express*, July 8, 2016; https://www.express.co.uk/life-style/life/687631/Women-comfortable-with-themselves-this-age.

28. Jeanna Bryner, "Does Old Age Bring Happiness or Despair?" *LiveScience*, April 4, 2010; https://www.livescience.com/6274-age-bring-happiness-despair.html.

29. Jim McCormick, *The Power of Risk* (San Francisco, CA: Maxwell Press, 2008), p. 146.

30. Ibid., p. 147.

31. Jonathan J. Rolison, Yaniv Hanoch, Stacey Wood, and Pi-Ju Liu, "Risk-Taking Differences Across the Adult Life Span: A Question of Age and Domain," *The Journals of Gerontology: Series B*, October 2013; Volume 69, Issue 6; 870–80; https://academic.oup.com/psychsocgerontology/article/69/6/870/545646.

32. Carolyn Dean, MD, *Menopause Naturally* (New York: McGraw-Hill Education, 1999), p. 4.

33. R. C. Bump, W. G. Hurt, J. A. Fantl, and J. F. Wyman, "Assessment of Kegel Pelvic Muscle Exercise Performance after Brief Verbal Instruction," *American Journal of Obstetrics and Gynecology*, 1991; Volume 165, Issue 2; 322–29.

34. From an email sent by Brent Reider, September 16, 2018, with explicit permission of "Hilary," the person providing the testimonial.

35. Interview with Brent Reider, September 16, 2018.

Glossary of Terms Related to Menopause and Intimacy

Acupuncture—A pain-relief therapy and treatment involving the use of fine needles inserted into targeted areas of the body; documented potential to relief hot flashes

Adenosine triphosphate (ATP)—The body's direct energy supply

Amygdala—A bit of gray matter that is part of the limbic system of the brain; it is involved in the experiencing of emotions (*See also* Limbic system)

Androgen—A male sex hormone such as testosterone (*See also* Testosterone)

Androgen therapy—The administration of testosterone for medical reasons; in menopausal women, used to treat symptoms such as low sexual desire, low sexual satisfaction, fatigue, and depression

Bioidentical hormones—Hormones identical in molecular structure to those women make in their bodies; not found in this form in nature but are made, or synthesized, from plants

Cheesecake of Pleasure—Sex therapist Dr. Jenni Skyler's term for a variety of pleasure-focused activities that couples can enjoy

Clitoral complex—The external and internal portions of the clitoris consisting of the glans, or the small circular mass that is the visible part of the clitoral complex; the prepuce, also commonly called "the hood," which is the skin likened to the penile foreskin; the frenulum, a posterior fold; the body, which are two masses of erectile tissue; the bulbs, also called the clitoral vestibules; and two crura, which are two pieces of erectile tissue that surround the urethra

DOing—Refers to Deliberate Orgasm, a term and technique coined by The Welcomed Consensus to describe a pleasure-focused experience with emphasis on stroking the clitoris

Dopamine—A chemical that functions as a neurotransmitter in the brain; high dopamine levels mean you are in tune with pleasure, whereas reduced dopamine levels mean that your perceptions of reward and pleasure are low

Endorphins—A naturally produced opioid, meaning they help us handle pain and can produce a "high"; the physical stress of exercise gets endorphins going in the system

Erotic intelligence—As defined by psychotherapist and sexuality expert Esther Perel (*Mating in Captivity: Unlocking Erotic Intelligence*), a state of being that has more to do with imagination than something primal and animalistic; it is rooted in curiosity, playfulness, and mystery

Estradiol—The form of estrogen that decreases at menopause

Estrogen—Steroid hormones that promote development and maintenance of female characteristics

Extragenital matrix—Developed by Drs. Beverly Whipple and Gina Ogden, it is a table to help women and men discover areas of sensual and sexual pleasure as well as what kind of non-genital touching makes a person feel good

Flibanserin—A drug to improve female sex drive; it raises levels of dopamine and norepinephrine while it reduces the amount of serotonin in the body; developed to treat hypoactive sexual desire disorder

G spot—Short for Gräfenberg spot; once thought to be a distinct anatomical structure, but properly identified by Drs. Beverly Whipple (*The G Spot*) and John Perry as an internal area of sensation related to clitoral arousal

Hippocampus—Part of the limbic system; puts the puzzle pieces of short-term memory together to give us long-term memories (*See also* Limbic system)

Hormone therapy (HT) (*aka* hormone replacement therapy)—Use of synthetic and/or bioidentical hormones to make up for the loss of female hormones during menopause, and potentially afterward

Hyaluronic acid—A natural substance found in the body's connective, neural, and epithelial tissues that is used in some vaginal moisturizers as well as facial rejuvenation products

Hypothalamus—A region of the brain that links the nervous and endocrine systems and controls the pituitary gland; key in controlling body temperature, thirst, and hunger, among other basic functions, and is involved in sleep and emotions

Isoflavones—Plant sources of estrogen (*See also* Phytoestrogens)

Kegels (pronounced *Kay*-gils)—Exercises for the pelvic floor developed by Arnold Kegel, an American gynecologist

Libido—The biological component of sexual feelings; the animal desire for sex

Lichen sclerosus—An autoimmune attack on the vulva that causes a thinning of the tissues, fissuring, itching, and burning

Limbic system—Part of the brain that emerged with mammals; associated with desires, emotions, and memory

Lubricants (*aka* lubes)—Oil-based, water-based, or silicone-based substances used to treat the dryness in the vulvar and vaginal areas that is a source of painful sex

Menopause—Phase of life in which menstrual cycles permanently cease due to the depletion of eggs in the ovaries; a result of aging unless induced through disease, trauma, or treatments for disease or trauma

Neocortex—Part of the brain called the neomammalian complex or "primate brain"; responsible for language, imagination, learning, and consciousness

Neurotransmitter—A chemical transmitting nerve impulses from one spot to another; some neurotransmitters also fall into the category of hormone

Oxytocin—Hormone most associated with loving touch; enhances the desire for interpersonal closeness and amplifies feelings of empathy; produced in the hypothalamus and secreted into the bloodstream by the pituitary gland

Parathyroid gland—Regulates the blood's calcium levels

Pelvic floor—The base of muscles attached to the pelvis that is the "ground floor" of the abdomen

Pelvic organ prolapse—Serious weakness in muscles supporting the uterus, bladder, and rectum allowing one or more of the pelvic organs to drop or press into or out of the vagina

Perimenopause—The phase of life when the number of eggs in the ovaries has dropped to a very low level and the body is transitioning to the end of reproductive years

Peripheral serotonin—Serotonin made in the digestive tract

Phytoestrogens—Plant sources of estrogen (*See also* Isoflavones)

Pituitary glands—Control other endocrine glands and regulate processes including growth, blood pressure, and water balance

Probiotics—Live microorganisms that confer a beneficial effect when taken in adequate and appropriate amounts

Progesterone—A steroid hormone that stimulates the uterus to prepare for reproduction

Progestin—Synthetic progesterone

Reptilian complex—Part of the brain controlling involuntary survival functions, such as heart rate and breathing and fight-or-flight responses to a threat; reproduction is part of survival

Selective serotonin reuptake inhibitors (SSRIs)—Antidepressants sometimes prescribed for menopausal women to reduce the severity and frequency of hot flashes (*See also* Serotonin-norepinephrine uptake inhibitors)

Sensate focus—The foundation of the sex therapy developed by William Masters and Virginia Johnson; it is designed to help participants focus on their sensory perceptions and sensuality instead of goal-oriented behavior

Sensual researcher—A term used by The Welcomed Consensus instructors to describe someone who methodically determines what feels pleasurable to herself

Serotonin—The "sunshine hormone," meaning that it engenders a feel-good sense; also production is triggered by sunshine, among other environmental as well as dietary factors

Serotonin-norepinephrine uptake inhibitors (SNRIs)—Antidepressants sometimes prescribed for menopausal women to reduce the severity and frequency of hot flashes (*See also* Selective serotonin reuptake inhibitors)

Serotonin syndrome—A group of symptoms that may follow use of certain menopause and antidepressant medications that affect serotonin levels in the body; the symptoms may include changes in mental status, coordination problems, racing heartbeat, sweating, nausea or diarrhea, and a number of other problems (*See also* Selective serotonin reuptake inhibitors *and* Serotonin-norepinephrine uptake inhibitors)

Sexual motivation—The psychological drive to be physical, emotional, and intimate with another person

Surgical menopause—Menopause induced by surgical removal of ovaries or by damage to them from radiation, chemotherapy, medication, or other trauma

Synthetic hormones—Chemical substances produced in laboratories that are supposed to mimic the function of hormones produced by the body; they differ in structure from the naturally occurring hormones

Testosterone—A steroid hormone, which in a woman is produced in the ovaries and adrenal cortex; known as the male sex hormone, it has a key role in libido (*See also* Libido)

Thyroid gland—Produces hormones such as thyroxine that controls energy-related reactions and other functions in cells

Vasomotor symptoms—Menopause symptoms related to fluctuations in body temperature resulting in hot flashes, night sweats, and flushes

Vulvovaginal atrophy (*aka* vaginal atrophy)—A result of decreased estrogen that shows up as dryness in the vagina and external area, as well as thinning of the vaginal walls and loss of elasticity; a major cause of painful intercourse that can be countered with a variety of effective treatments

Index

About the Author

Maryann Karinch is the author of thirty books, including *Sex and Cancer: Intimacy, Love, and Romance after Diagnosis and Treatment* with Saketh Guntupalli (Rowman & Littlefield, 2017). Maryann has teamed up with seven doctors, two interrogators, a former CIA operative, and several other experts to produce some of the books in her list. She is an American Council on Exercise (ACE)–certified personal trainer. Among the international media outlets that have covered Maryann's human behavior work are: ABC News; *Boston Globe*; *Christian Science Monitor*; *Dallas Morning News*; *Fast Company*; *Huffington Post*; *Washington Post*; *New York Daily News*; NPR, and others.